Dyslexia: a hundred years on

Dyslexia: a hundred years on

T.R. Miles
and
Elaine Miles

Open University Press
Milton Keynes · Philadelphia

Open University Press
Celtic Court
22 Ballmoor
Buckingham
MK18 1XW

and
1900 Frost Road, Suite 101
Bristol, PA 19007, USA

First Published 1990

British Library Cataloguing in Publication Data

Miles, T.R. (Thomas Richard), 1923–
  Dyslexia: a hundred years on
  1. Man. Dyslexia
  I. Title   II. Miles, Elaine
  616.8553

  ISBN 0-335-09541-0
  ISBN 0-335-09540-2 pbk

Library of Congress Cataloging-in-Publication Data

Miles, T.R. (Thomas Richard)
  Dyslexia: a hundred years on/by T.R. Miles and Elaine Miles.
      p.   cm.
  Includes bibliographical references.
  ISBN 0-335-09541-0: ISBN 0-335-09540-2 (pbk.)
  1. Dyslexia.   I. Miles, Elaine.   II. Title.
  [DNLM: 1. Dyslexia. WM 475 M643da]
  RC394.W6M55 1990
  616.85'53--dc20
  DNLM/DLC
  for Library of Congress   90-7088 CIP

Typeset by GCS, Leighton Buzzard, Beds.
Printed in Great Britain by J.W. Arrowsmith Ltd, Bristol

Contents

Preface

It is nearly 100 years since Pringle Morgan (1896) first published his famous account of Percy, a boy of 14 who could 'only with difficulty spell out words of one syllable', who wrote his name as 'Precy' and 'did not notice the mistake until his attention was called to it more than once'. Yet 'the schoolmaster who taught him for some years says that he would be the smartest lad in the school if the instruction were entirely oral' (p. 1378).

In calling this book *Dyslexia: a hundred years on* our intention has been to review some of the more important changes which have taken place in the dyslexia field over this 100 years. During the last decade in particular the literature on reading and language difficulties has increased massively, and it follows that a comprehensive review of all of it – even if we were capable of undertaking such a mammoth task! – would almost certainly have made the book unreadable. Instead, we have selected a restricted number of studies which we regard as interesting and important and which we then discuss in varying degrees of detail.

Although we have tried to present the research fairly, we can make no claims to impartiality in the choice of material chosen. In our judgement the evidence points unequivocally in a particular direction, viz. that there are some individuals who display an anomaly of development which results in weakness at the *phonological* level, that is, in using speech sounds in a language system. The so-called 'classic signs' of dyslexia can on our view properly be called a 'syndrome' (that is, a cluster of symptoms which are regularly found together), and we believe them to be the consequences of this phonological weakness. This syndrome has been described by Critchley (1970) as 'specific developmental dyslexia' (in contrast with 'dyslexia' *simpliciter*). His claim (1970, p. 11) is that there is 'a specific type of developmental dyslexia occurring in the midst of but nosologically apart from the *olla podrida* of bad readers'. (According to the dictionary '*olla podrida*' is a kind of Spanish stew containing many varieties of ingredient!) In our opinion Critchley's views on dyslexia are basically correct.

A central problem throughout the book has been that of terminology. Pringle Morgan and Hinshelwood spoke of 'word blindness' and Orton of 'strephosymbolia'; and in the literature, besides 'specific developmental dyslexia', one finds 'developmental aphasia', 'legasthenia', 'specific reading difficulty', 'specific learning disability', and many other descriptions. Although in using these expressions people may well have been speaking about broadly similar children, the matter is not simply one of interchangeable synonyms. There is, in the words of Naidoo (1972, p. 8), 'a multiplicity of notions about the characteristics and aetiology of the disorders they describe'. Whatever expression one chooses, therefore, one is open to the accusation of seeming to be begging important questions. This seems to us unavoidable; and we can only alert the reader to the fact that we are approaching the subject from the point of view which, over the years, has seemed to us the most helpful one.

It will be seen throughout the book that those whose research is reported have by no means been unanimous in their terminology. Some of them have described their subjects as 'dyslexic' while implying only that they had severe, or unexpectedly severe, reading problems (for instance, Vellutino 1979; Stein and Fowler 1985, and the numerous researchers into acquired reading disorder); some, perhaps wishing to avoid unnecessary theoretical commitment, have spoken of 'backward readers' (for instance, Bryant and Bradley 1985); while some have deliberately described their subjects as 'dyslexic' with the explicit intention of talking about 'specific developmental dyslexia' (for instance, Hallgren 1950; Naidoo 1972; Miles 1983; and Thomson 1984). In most cases, though by no means all, the researchers have in fact used largely similar selection procedures, subjects being chosen for special study because there was evidence of a discrepancy between their reading level and their intelligence level as judged by standard intelligence tests. However, this does not by itself justify the assumption that 'dyslexics', or whatever else one calls them, picked out in this way, are a homogeneous group or that generalizations about the 'typical' dyslexic can be made without further argument. This is an issue which cannot be decided until one has reviewed a large quantity of research. Meanwhile our general policy will be to follow wherever possible the terminology of the original researcher (for example, by using 'reading disabled' if the original researcher used this expression), but otherwise to use the terms 'dyslexia' and 'dyslexic' unless there is good reason for not doing so. Those reading this book will then need to decide for themselves to what extent generalization is justified.

There is yet another complication in that those who have studied 'specific developmental dyslexia' usually argue that the condition can be present even when reading skills are adequate (Critchley 1970; Naidoo 1972; Miles 1987). If this is correct there is no contradiction in saying that a person is dyslexic while nevertheless being a competent reader; and, indeed, many dyslexic adults come in this category. When this issue arises the important thing is to note how the subjects in a particular experiment were selected.

On the few occasions where it has been necessary to refer to unspecified individuals in the singular we have used 'he'/'his' and 'she'/'her' at random. Although there are in fact more dyslexic boys than girls (see Chapter 6), what we have to say applies to individuals of either sex.

We are grateful to all those who have helped us with the writing of this book, in particular Dr Pauline Horne, Dr Gordon Brown and Professor Phillip Williams. Responsibility for all errors, however, must remain with the authors.

T.R.M.
E.M.

Acknowledgements

Special thanks are due to Educators Publishing Service, Inc. of Cambridge, Mass., for permission to quote from the Gillingham Stillman manual and to W.M. Freeman of New York for permission to quote from Springer and Deutsch.

1

The genesis of an idea

By the middle of the nineteenth century it had come to be recognized that injury to the brain could sometimes result in disorders of thought and speech. These disorders are known as the *aphasias*, where by derivation 'aphasia' means literally 'not speaking'.

A graphic account of the early history of aphasia will be found in Head (1926). Here, by way of illustration, is a description which he quotes from an account by Franz Joseph Gall (1758–1828) of a patient whom we would now call 'aphasic'.

> His mind ('esprit') found the answer to questions addressed to him and he carried out all he was told to do; shown an arm-chair and asked if he knew what it was he answered by seating himself in it. He could not articulate on the spot a word pronounced for him to repeat; but a few moments later the word escaped from his lips as if involuntarily.
>
> (Head 1926, p. 10)

This observation is perhaps the more noteworthy since posterity thinks of Gall not as a writer on aphasia but as a crank who tried to relate personality characteristics to the shape of the person's skull! It is interesting that 'phrenology', the name given to this kind of enquiry, has turned out to be a blind alley, whereas the study of aphasia has not.

The distinction between the voluntary and automatic use of words came to the fore in the work of Hughlings Jackson (see Taylor 1931, for an edited version of his writings).

Coining the word 'verbalising' to include all the modes in which words serve, we see that there are two great divisions or rather extremes of verbalising: one is the voluntary use of words (speech); the other is the automatic use of words.

(Taylor 1931, p. 65)

Jackson goes on to point out that the words 'yes' and 'no' are often only of 'interjectional' value.

Curiously we find that the patient who can *reply* 'No' correctly may be quite unable to *say* 'no' when told.... He may utter oaths or other ejaculations when excited which he cannot *say* – cannot repeat – when he tries to do so. He may say 'Thanks' or 'Good-bye' on fit occasions but not when he tries.... He may be unable to put out his tongue when he tries but move it well in all automatic operations.

(Taylor 1931, p. 65)

'Speech' is used by Jackson to mean 'voluntary speech'. Speech in this sense is necessary for purposeful writing.

It is a great mistake to suppose that a speechless patient can write, that is, write in the sense of expressing himself, because he can sign his name or because he can copy what is put before him.... When we write we merely translate nascently revived words into written symbols. We have to speak 'inside ourselves' first.

(Taylor 1931, p. 20)

The same holds in the case of reading:

The speechless man cannot read, not even to himself. It is not that his eyes, or rather the parts of his brain which contain processes for the recognition of images of things, are affected, for he does recognise objects, and when he cannot read can recognise headings ... The difficulty is still one of loss of speech. Written and printed words strictly have no meaning. They are merely arbitrary signs of words. They require translation into words and into an *order* of words.... The speechless man is not wordless; his defect is that he cannot revive words *voluntarily*.

(Taylor 1931, p. 20)

The distinction between 'voluntary' and 'automatic' has its basis, Jackson believes, in the differences of function between the two cerebral hemispheres:

The fact of most significance is, not that disease of the *left* hemisphere mostly makes a man speechless, but that disease of but *one* hemisphere can make him speechless. I have suggested that one hemisphere is for the automatic, and the other for the voluntary and automatic, use of words.

(Taylor 1931, p. 73)

The notion of *balance* between the two cerebral hemispheres has turned out to be of fundamental importance, and we shall be referring to it again in Chapter 3. In 1861 it was claimed by P.P. Broca that aphasia in a particular patient 'was the result of a profound but accurately circumscribed lesion of the posterior third of the second and third frontal convolutions' (Head 1926, p. 25). This particular area has subsequently been designated 'Broca's area'. Even at the time, however, it was recognized that the attempt to locate speech functions in a few restricted areas in the brain was an over-simplification; and it is interesting that, in a paper written over a century later, the author concludes that 'none of the theories of the various types of aphasia has had general acceptance. In spite of a century of study, the mechanisms of speech and language disorders remain as challenging problems' (Richardson 1989, p. 5).

Shortly after Broca's discovery Kussmaul (1878) introduced the concepts of 'word deafness' and 'word blindness' (*surditas et caecitas verbalis*). These are his original words (pp. 772–3):

> Patients who suffer from word deafness and possess at the same time the ability to express themselves in words, but use many words in the wrong places, and often distort them, leave on the minds of the observers the impression that they are crazed.

He later points out (p. 774) that such patients are not genuinely deaf, since they 'perceive and pay attention to calls, noises, and murmurs'. Similarly: 'A complete text-blindness may exist even though the power of sight, the intellect, and the power of speech are intact' (p. 775). In support he cites observations by colleagues, for instance of a woman of 45 who 'saw the text, distinguished the forms of the letters, and could even copy the text, but was incapable of translating the words into spoken words and thoughts' (p. 776). In another case a patient 'lost entirely the power to read printing and writing. He saw the text but did not understand it ... His conversation was good ... but occasionally the names of streets, persons, and things failed him' (p. 776).

It was then only a short step to the view that there could be a congenital form of word blindness which might explain diffi-culties in learning to read in apparently intelligent children. Here

is some further information about Percy, the boy referred to in
the Preface:

> Percy F... has always been a bright and intelligent boy, quick at
> games, and in no way inferior to others of his age. His great
> difficulty has been – and is now – his inability to learn to read. This
> inability is so remarkable, and so pronounced, that I have no doubt
> it is due to some congenital defect.... In spite of ... laborious and
> persistent training, he can only with difficulty spell out words of
> one syllable.

> (Morgan 1896, p. 1378)

There follows an account of some of his spelling errors. They
included a mistake over his own name, 'Precy' for 'Percy', as well
as 'scone for 'song', 'soojock' for 'subject', and 'seasow' for
'seashore'. He was able to recognize the words 'and', 'the' and 'of',
and (surprisingly, in the light of recent knowledge) was able to do
a complicated multiplication sum. In contrast:

> Other words he never seems to remember, no matter how
> frequently he may have met them. He seems to have no power of
> preserving and storing up the visual impression produced by
> words – hence the words, though seen, have no significance for
> him. His visual memory for words is defective or absent; which is
> equivalent to saying that he is what Kussmaul has termed 'word
> blind' (*caecitas syllabaris et verbalis*).... It will be interesting to see
> what effect further training will have on his condition. His father
> informs me that the greatest difficulty was found in teaching the
> boy his letters, and they thought he never would learn them. No
> doubt he was originally letter blind (*caecitas litteralis*), but by dint of
> constant application this defect has been overcome.

During the next two decades the concept of 'congenital word
blindness' was given considerable prominence in the medical
literature as a result of the writings of James Hinshelwood, a
Glasgow eye surgeon. (For a detailed account of his views and a
list of earlier publications, see Hinshelwood 1917.) He had
already stated in 1900:

> I have little doubt that these cases of congenital word blindness
> are by no means so rare as the absence of recorded cases would
> lead us to infer. Their rarity is, I think, accounted for by the fact
> that when they do occur they are not recognised. It is a matter of
> the highest importance to recognise the cause and true nature of
> this difficulty in learning to read which is experienced by these
> children, otherwise they may be harshly treated as imbeciles or

incorrigibles, and either neglected or punished for a defect for which they are in no wise responsible.

(Hinshelwood 1917, pp. 42–3)

His account of the term is as follows:

By the term congenital word blindness, we mean a congenital defect occurring in children with otherwise normal and un-damaged brains characterised by a difficulty in learning to read so great that it is manifestly due to a pathological condition, and where the attempts to teach the child by the ordinary methods have completely failed.

(Hinshelwood 1917, p. 40)

This is a strong statement, and its repercussions have remained with us right up to the present time.

Hinshelwood also noted that the condition could sometimes be hereditary (1917, Chapter 3) and (p. 53) that it was more common in boys than in girls. He was also in no doubt that the children could be helped even though this required considerable effort. His views on teaching will be referred to in Chapter 10.

The last of the early pioneers to be discussed in this chapter will be the American neurologist, Samuel Orton. Orton believed, like Hinshelwood, that our understanding of developmental language disorders in children could be greatly increased if we took into account the acquired disorders of the adult. He differed from him, however, in respect of terminology. In particular he suggested (Orton 1937, p. 71) that the term 'congenital word blindness' is misleading, since 'there is no true blindness in the ordinary sense of the term nor, indeed, is there even blindness for words'. What he specially noted was 'a striking tendency to distorted order in the recall of letters shown in the attempts of these children to read a word or to spell it'. He therefore proposed the term 'strephosymbolia' (literally 'twisting of symbols') as a more informative description than 'word blindness'. He believed that the condition often ran in families and that among affected persons and their relatives there were sometimes unusual patterns of handedness and eyedness.

Studies of laterality in cases of developmental alexia have shown a very considerable number of crossed patterns between handed-ness and eyedness ... but this is by no means without exception and we have encountered extreme cases of the reading disability in children who were right sided.... The family history in by far the great majority of cases shows the presence of left-handedness in the stock.

(Orton 1937, p. 90)

According to Orton difficulties over ordering could take various forms. There could be transpositions in spoken language, for example 'button cuffs' for 'cuff buttons' or 'emeny' for 'enemy'. Above all there were what he called 'reversals'. The following is his account of the matter:

> The reversals are of two types. First, those in which confusion exists between the letters with the same form but opposite orientation, as when b is confused with d, and p with q. These we have called static reversals. The second is when there is an element of sinistrad progression through a series of letters as when *was* is read as *saw*, or *tomorrow* as *tworrom*. These we have called kinetic reversals. The two types are practically always to be found associated in any case of strephosymbolia. The frequency with which errors by reversal appeared in the work of a given case proved to correlate with the amount of his retardation in reading.

(Orton 1937, p. 150)

Sadly, no figures are given by which one could check this last statement, and his evidence for family sinistrality (Orton 1966, p. 145) is by no means decisive.

His account of the neurological basis of strephosymbolia is as follows:

> It is evident in the untrained mirror reading skill shown by some strephosymbolics that during attempts to learn to read words in the dextrad direction the brain has registered these words in the sinistrad position as well, so that they have become serviceable for recognition of the mirrored copy, and similarly in certain cases of the special writing disability... the brain has received and registered the mirrored forms with such fidelity that mirror writing of a very acceptable quality has been possible with no instruction and no practice. [In normal readers] any registrations which may have occurred in the non-dominant hemisphere have been elided or are unused.

(Orton 1937, pp. 151–2)

It was Orton who, along with Anna Gillingham, pioneered a systematic teaching programme aimed specifically at children with these problems (see Chapter 10); and it is interesting that he was also fully aware of the feelings of inferiority which could arise after repeated failure (Orton 1937, p. 135). He was clearly a

person of wide-ranging intellectual curiosity as well as being a
very sensitive observer.

Both Hinshelwood and Orton are now respected as great
pioneers, and rightly so. In the light of more recent knowledge,
however, it is perhaps justified to offer some critical comments.
It is, of course, quite possible for an investigator to discover a
new phenomenon or propose an important fresh classification
and yet to use terminology which has misleading theoretical
associations.

In this case it is no surprise to find that Hinshelwood, an eye
surgeon, discussing the problems with other eye specialists in
ophthalmological journals, should regard them as essentially
visual in character. For example, he writes: 'The defect in these
children is then a strictly specialised one, *viz.* a difficulty in
acquiring and storing up in the brain the *visual memories* of words
and letters' (our italics) (Hinshelwood 1917, p. 52). Orton, too,
despite his opposition to the term 'word blindness', was still
thinking in visuo-spatial terms: the letters were the wrong way
round or in the wrong order in respect of their *visual appearance.*

Now it is of course true that when one looks at children's
misspellings the letters are *soon* to be the wrong way round or in
reverse order. This, however, does not of itself entitle us to say
that the problem is a visual one. Orton assumes, perhaps rather
simplistically, that events in the world are mapped on to the
visual areas of the brain in the form of a simple one-one
correspondence – a view that had already been challenged by the
Gestalt psychologists (see Koffka 1935, pp. 96, 97, 117) and was
later submitted to devastating criticism by Gibson (1968). Only if
such an assumption were justified would it make sense to
postulate non-elision of 'engrams' in the brain as the explanation
of 'strephosymbolia'.

This emphasis on vision generated a wide range of 'visual'
terms. Not only were children described as 'word blind', but a
'Word Blind Institute' was set up in Copenhagen and a 'World
Blind Centre' in London. When 'b' and 'd' were confused people
spoke of 'reversals', of 'mirror writing', and of 'mirror images';
and terminology of this sort coloured popular conceptions of
dyslexia for many years to come. Even Orton's carefully drawn
distinction between 'static' and 'kinetic' reversals was sometimes
overlooked: 'b' is indeed the mirror image of 'd' but it is plain from
simple optics that 'was' is not the mirror image of 'saw'!

It is particularly informative to look at his list of 'typical examples of misspellings due to kinetic reversals' (Orton 1966, p. 181). These include: 'wram' for 'warm', 'inght' for 'night', 'gril' for 'girl', 'hte' for 'the', 'ieght' for 'eight', 'Jhon' for 'John', 'rophan' for 'orphan', and 'theet' for 'teeth'. Twenty misspellings are cited in all; and it is noteworthy that in eight cases the error consists in the transposition of an 'r' and a vowel. Now such transpositions are a common feature in the historical development of oral language; for example, 'griddle' and 'girdle' are alternative versions of the same word. However, the fact that such transpositions can occur in oral language suggests that they cannot simply be due to mistakes over the visual appearance of the word in its written form. There is in any case an alternative explanation. Instead of supposing that the child has moved through the word from right to left instead of from left to right, one possibility is that he vaguely remembered that certain letters are present but that because of a memory limitation he was unable to put them down in the right order. It is a further limitation of the 'strephosymbolia' theory that it does not explain why there should be left–right confusions rather than up–down ones or why the confusions should be restricted to symbols and not occur in the case of familiar objects.

Later research has cast doubt on the value of this predominantly visual approach. In its place there has been a shift towards what can be called a 'language-based' approach. This change of emphasis will be discussed further in Chapters 6 and 9. Meanwhile it can be said of both Hinshelwood and Orton that though their theories now seem highly questionable the observations which they made are of lasting importance.

2

Problems of method

Dyslexia has 'many faces' (Rawson 1986), and a variety of different procedures have been used for studying it. In the chapters which follow we shall be selecting for discussion some of the more important of these studies. As a preliminary, however, we thought it would be useful to make some comments on problems of method. Our purpose in doing so is to help the reader to evaluate the varied (and sometimes conflicting) claims about dyslexia which are found in the literature.

We shall begin by saying something about research methods in general, after which we shall call attention to some of the precautions which need to be observed in dyslexia research if erroneous conclusions are to be avoided. What we have to say relates primarily to psychological research, though some of it may have applicability in other fields.

Research methods can usefully be classified under three heads, viz. (i) individual case histories, (ii) group comparisons, and (iii) comparisons of the same individual in different conditions (single-subject designs). No one of these methods should be regarded as the only correct one; each has its value and its limitations, and one or another may be appropriate according to one's purposes.

Individual case histories, both in the study of dyslexia and elsewhere, are often of particular value as a starting point. They suggest topics for further investigation and set the stage for research of a more systematic kind. The importance of informal observation has not always been adequately recognized. In psychology especially, before one starts to investigate a particular topic it is usually wise to get the 'feel' of the situation by talking to individuals and obtaining an overall picture; and in the case of dyslexia research this involves getting to know individual dyslexics. Only later should one be thinking in terms of systematic comparisons. Some psychologists speak disparagingly of 'anecdotal evidence', that is, accounts of events which allegedly happened but at no specified time and with no corroborative detail. A carefully documented case history, however, need not be 'anecdotal' in this bad sense; one of its important functions is to suggest hypotheses which can later be tested more systematically. It can also contribute towards securing what has been called 'ecological validity'; that is, it can point to conclusions which hold good outside the restricted environment of the psychology laboratory. Case histories can also act as a check if, as sometimes happens, researchers who have met only a few dyslexics ask inappropriate questions or draw questionable conclusions. In contrast an experienced teacher, after seeing individual children over many years, is often in a position to make entirely valid generalizations, and to correct them if later events show that they are mistaken, even though such a person would not pretend to be doing systematic research.

The main limitations of the case history method are twofold. In the first place there may be dangers in trying to generalize from one case to another; thus, if a particular dyslexic individual behaves in some particularly striking way it is difficult to be sure whether it would be right to expect the same thing in another dyslexic. Secondly, there is no way of establishing whether one occurrence is the cause of another. Thus if a poor reader receives teaching by a particular method and her reading improves there can at best be presumptive evidence of a causal connection between the method and the improvement. A more subtle design would be needed, and it would be necessary to exclude other explanations, for instance that the improvement was the result of increased confidence or, indeed, simply due to normal processes of development.

The method of group comparison arose originally as an attempt to overcome these limitations. It is by far the most commonly used of research designs, and it takes a variety of forms. The basic pattern is the comparison of an experimental group with a control group.

The following will serve as an example. If one wishes to find out if a particular task – say producing the names of colours at speed – is difficult for dyslexics one would take a group of dyslexics and compare them with suitably matched non-dyslexics. It would be necessary to specify how the dyslexics were picked out (that is, provide an 'operational definition' of 'dyslexic', so that one is in effect saying 'By a "dyslexic" person is meant someone who satisfied these particular criteria'), and it would also be necessary to ensure that the non-dyslexics were like the dyslexics in all relevant ways apart from not being dyslexic. If this last precaution is not taken, then any differences between the two groups may not be anything to do with the dyslexia as such but could have arisen because the non-dyslexics were older, more intelligent, from a different social background, and so on. In addition, each subject in the experiment needs to be treated in a strictly standardized way; for example, if in this case the colours to be named were presented on a card, this card would need to be the same for everyone and the instructions would need to be the same; otherwise all kinds of uncontrolled factors may influence the results. There is also the problem of generalizing. If there are differences between a group of, say, fifteen 10-year-old dyslexics and fifteen matched non-dyslexics, it is not self-evident that one can immediately generalize from this result to *all* dyslexics. The extent to which generalization is possible may depend on the particular circumstances of the experiment.

In many contexts it is necessary to use statistical techniques. A common use for these techniques (though there are many others) is to determine what is called the 'significance level' of the results – that is, the degree of confidence one can have that the observed differences are genuine and not just the result of a chance fluctuation on this particular occasion. In the discussions which follow we shall not make any reference to significance levels; but these levels will normally be found in the original research papers.

Somewhat less well known are *single-subject* designs. One of the limitations of the group comparison method is that it does not do full justice to the fact of individual variability. It may be that the mean (average) score for a group of individuals on a particular test is so-and-so, and one can, of course, work out statistical measures, such as the standard deviation, which indicate how widely the scores are scattered around the mean. In some contexts, however, variability is of interest in its own right, and when this is the case single-subject comparisons are desirable.

The basic difference between a group design and a single-subject design is that in the first case one gives a standard task to a large number of subjects, while in the second one successively gives different tasks to the same subject. In some experiments, with either humans or animals, it is possible in a single-subject design to check in the first place on what the subject typically does without any intervention at all (baseline phase), and then study the effect of introducing some new treatment. In the right context one can be reasonably confident of a causal connection between the new treatment and the changes in behaviour.

It remains to consider various safeguards that are necessary in dyslexia research. One of the most important of these is to make sure that suitable control groups are introduced. Thus if one simply compares poor readers with normal readers and finds differences (for example that the poor readers have a short memory span for auditorily presented digits), it is impossible to say whether these differences are the cause of the poor reading, its effect, or neither. It is now widely recognized that an important safeguard in many contexts is to compare dyslexics not only with age-matched non-dyslexics but with younger dyslexics matched for reading age. If differences are still found, these cannot be due to lack of reading experience as such. Of course if on a particular task dyslexics are *on a level* with chronological-age-matched controls then a reading-age-matched control group is unnecessary (for further discussion of this point, see Bryant and Bradley 1985).

Another important safeguard is to control for what is called the 'Hawthorne effect'. This term arose as a result of work carried out at the Hawthorne plant in the USA in the late 1920s (for sources, see Sprott 1952). What appears to have happened is that a routine investigation was carried out to see if productivity would be improved if the lighting conditions were made better. It did – but it did so again when the level of illumination was reduced to below what it had originally been! It therefore came to be believed, probably with justification, that it was not the changes in lighting as such which caused the improved output, but the fact that the employees realized that someone was interested in their working conditions. In general, the expression 'Hawthorne effect' is used in any situation where a result occurs not for the reasons originally intended but because of improved morale when something new has been tried.

Closely related to the Hawthorne effect is what is called the 'placebo effect'. It has long been recognized by medical researchers that medication can sometimes produce good effects not because of the chemical properties of the medicine but because patients *believed* that they would benefit.

It should be noted that Hawthorne effects and placebo effects are not bad in themselves. It is perfectly justified to provide a particular kind of teaching or treatment even if one does not fully know why it works; and if, for all one knows, the beliefs of the pupil or the patient are a contributory factor in bringing about success, this is a bonus and not a thing to be regretted. Those doing research, however, need to be careful, since their task is to tease out what different causal factors are at work; and if they do not control for Hawthorne and placebo effects they will mislead themselves. This 'teasing out' is an essential feature of scientific method. To make the corn grow it may be efficacious to sprinkle water on it and say 'abracadabra'; but it is only if one follows the scientific principle of varying only one condition at a time that one will learn that the sprinkling of the water is essential to the outcome whereas the saying of 'abracadabra' is not.

In the case of dyslexia it is particularly important that those who claim that a particular teaching method is effective should not mislead themselves. It is always a wise precaution to ask, 'To what extent is the success due to the teaching method as such and to what extent could it be due to the personality of the teacher or the novelty of the situation?' A possible safeguard is to arrange for different teachers to use the same method; then, if there is success with more than one teacher, it is at least more likely that the method is the important factor. In practice, however, it is by no means easy to ensure that teachers are using methods that are genuinely the same or genuinely different, since it is very difficult to keep track of the many incidental things that they do. For example, a teacher who, as part of a research programme, is believed to be teaching by 'look and say' as opposed to phonic methods may pronounce a word extra slowly and thus unwittingly provide an indication of its phonic structure. It is also possible that the gestures and comments of an unsympathetic teacher may lead to less effective results even though the method itself is perfectly sound.

There are, of course, many alleged 'remedies' for dyslexia on the market; and while it is possible that some of them are useful even though their usefulness has not been adequately demonstrated, a knowledge of research methods is of great help in

evaluating them. In the absence of any statistical data one is right
to be suspicious; and even if statistics are produced it is wise to
submit them to critical scrutiny. It is possible, for instance, that
the authors may over-generalize from their results or may
mislead themselves as to the direction of causality. In this
connection readers may like to consult Wilsher and Taylor
(1986). This is a paper which deals harshly – but justly – with
claims to success which are unproven; and it provides a very good
introduction to the study of research methodology.

Finally, some safeguards should be mentioned in connection
with the interpretation of test results. In the case of reading tests
it is important to note whether the task calls for comprehension
or only for single-word recognition. In the case of both reading
and spelling tests careful examination of individual items is
usually essential; and there is particular danger in elaborate
statistical treatment of scores which even in their raw form were
of doubtful significance. There is a further danger in that in
many cases the scoring system is such that a correct response is
awarded a single point and nothing else is taken into account,
even though in practice it is usually very important to take note
both of 'near misses' and of the types of error made. In general
it should be remembered that two children may obtain the
same score on a test even though the kinds of mistake that
they are making are very different; and the inference that they
are at 'the same reading level' or 'the same spelling level' should
not be made uncritically.

There are even more problems in connection with the concept
of 'IQ'. It is of course useful, for both theoretical and practical
purposes, to be able to demonstrate that there are some tasks at
which dyslexics can be extremely successful. An IQ figure in the
traditional sense, however, represents the sum of a person's
performance on a wide range of different tasks; and it has been
found in the case of dyslexics (see Chapter 6) that some of the
components of these tasks are easy for them, others much more
difficult. Accounts of how dyslexics have behaved when given a
reading test, a spelling test, or an intelligence test are often very
informative; in contrast, inferences based solely on their 'scores'
should be treated with caution.

It is important to realize, whatever one's research field, that
conclusions may be correct even when they are not statistically
proven and that there is room for speculation even when
evidence is scanty. In the chapters which follow we shall try,

where possible, to indicate when we think a conclusion is well established and when we believe it to be more doubtful. The important thing, however, is not so much what we ourselves think, as that the reader should be able to make as informed a judgement as possible. Our aim in the present chapter has been to try to promote a greater awareness of what is required if research evidence is to be evaluated correctly.

3

Brain research

It will not be possible in the space of a brief chapter to provide any comprehensive account of the structures or functions of the human brain or to review the latest research in any detail. Our purpose in this chapter will rather be to try to convey the general tenor of some of this research in so far as it is relevant to dyslexia; and in particular we have had in mind the need to help the reader to distinguish what is well established from what is speculative or dubious.

As a general background for the understanding of research it is useful to think about the brain in evolutionary terms. One of the questions which came to the fore as a result in particular of the work of Charles Darwin was, 'How does a particular biological structure *benefit* the organism?' In the case of humans one may wonder at times how they survived at all! They are feebler than lions; they are slower at moving than deer or rabbits, and unlike wasps or jellyfish they cannot incapacitate their enemies by stinging them. Where they are distinctive, of course, is in the evolution of their brains; and it is because of their complex brain organization that they can emit a wide range of meaningful speech sounds and carry out delicate operations with their hands. There is no need for a 'sting' when one can render impotent the largest of animals by a poisoned arrow or by anaesthetic and pass on one's skills to one's descendants by means of language. Language, too, can help us to guide our behaviour by rules (Skinner 1969; Vygotski 1986), and, more than the members of any other species, we can take account of what is distant in both space and time. In view, therefore, of the overall importance of our ability to communicate with one another, it is worth while reflecting on the extreme complexity and delicacy of the mechanisms which make such communication possible. It is likely, as we shall see later in the book, that typical cases of dyslexia involve some disorder of the language function, and it is not altogether surprising from the biological point of view that these mechanisms should occasionally show minor flaws.

Anatomically the brain is divided into two halves (or 'hemispheres'), with dense collections of nerve cells (neurones) closely packed together inside the skull. The skull itself, of course, is no more than a protective covering, and it was a curious aberration on the part of certain nineteenth-century thinkers (the 'phrenologists') to suppose that the protrusions on the skull could be linked with personality characteristics (compare the reference to Gall in Chapter 1). The two cerebral hemispheres are approximately – though not exactly – symmetrical, as, indeed, are many other organs of the human body: in particular, we have two eyes, two ears, two nostrils, two arms and two legs, and, apart from a number of exceptions such as the heart and the liver, there are few bodily organs that are not found in duplicate.

Despite the relative similarity of the two cerebral hemispheres, however, it does not follow that they both carry out the same functions. Certain skills have become possible precisely because the hemispheres have *specialist* functions, one of them, usually the left, being distinctively involved in the production of language. This point has been confirmed by a number of different research techniques, and it may therefore be useful to give a brief review of the kinds of evidence which support this conclusion.

The Wada technique involves anaesthetizing one or other side of the brain by the injection of a drug, sodium amytal. The following account has been given by Springer and Deutsch (1984, pp. 20–1):

> Moments before the drug is injected the fully conscious patient lies flat on his or her back and is asked to count backward from 100 in threes. The patient is also asked to keep both arms raised in the air while counting. The drug is then slowly injected.... Within seconds of the injection dramatic results occur.
>
> First the area opposite to the side of the injection falls limp. Since each half of the brain controls the opposite half of the body, the falling arm tells the neurosurgeon that the drug has reached the proper hemisphere and has taken effect. Second, the patient

generally stops counting, either for a few seconds or for the duration of the drug's effect, depending on which hemisphere is affected. If the drug is injected on the same side as the hemisphere controlling speech, the patient remains speechless for 2 to 5 minutes, depending on the dose administered. If it is injected on the other side, the patient generally resumes counting within a few seconds and can answer questions with little difficulty while the drug is still inactivating the other half of the brain.

It is thus possible, by means of the Wada technique, to determine which side of the patient's brain controls speech, and this can be checked if an injection is given to the other side of the brain on another occasion. Use of the technique suggests that in the case of right-handers with no history of brain damage about 95 per cent have speech controlled by the left hemisphere. In the case of left-handers the figure is about 70 per cent, with 15 per cent having it controlled by the right hemisphere and 15 per cent having it controlled by both hemispheres.

Confirmation of these figures has come from a study (Russell and Espir 1961) of patients whose aphasia was due to bullet injuries. Of 189 right-handers 3 had entry wounds on the right and 186 on the left, while of 13 left-handers 4 had entry wounds on the right and 9 on the left.

For various medical reasons, particularly in the cases of acute epilepsy, it was sometimes thought helpful in the past to disconnect the two hemispheres by severing the corpus callosum, a bundle of centrally placed nerve fibres whose function is to relay signals from one half of the brain to the other. If patients who have undergone this form of surgery are presented with pictures of objects in the left visual field (so that impulses go to the right hemisphere), they are likely to have considerable difficulty in finding the names for these pictures, even though they are able to carry out a 'matching task', for example by feeling for the correct object from among several that are lying behind a screen out of sight. If the same pictures are presented to the left hemisphere, however, the patients will normally have no difficulty in finding the right name. This finding provides further support for the view that it is normally the left hemisphere, rather than the right, which is involved in the production of language.

Up to this point it has been possible to present reasonably 'hard' evidence. The precise role of the right hemisphere, however, is more uncertain. The commonly held view is that it is concerned with visuo-spatial tasks and that it processes information 'simultaneously and holistically' (Springer and Deutsch 1984, p. 45). It is also possible that many of the skills required for music are controlled from the right hemisphere (ibid., pp. 170–2), though not, of course, the skills in reading musical notation (compare Chapter 6 of this book).

In general it can be concluded that there is a body of firm knowledge about hemispheric specialization. We should like, however, to conclude this section of the chapter with a note of caution. For this purpose we cannot do better than quote some telling words of Springer and Deutsch (1984, p. 7):

> There has been a tendency to interpret every behavioral dichotomy, such as rational versus intuitive and deductive versus imaginative, in terms of left brain and right brain. This occupational hazard has been named 'dichotomania' by some. In addition, the dividing line between fact and fantasy has often been blurred, making it difficult for nonspecialists to know what is speculation and what has been established firmly as fact.

The BEAM technique (Brain Electrical Activity Mapping) is a development of the use of the electroencephalograph (EEG) and is a way of studying electrical activity in the brain. Another technique is PET-scan (Positron Emission Tomography), a technique by which it is possible to study cerebral metabolism, including blood flow in particular. Differences between dyslexics and controls have been reported in a number of studies, for instance Duffy *et al.* (1988), but no comprehensive theory has yet emerged. Those who wish to study the evidence in more detail may like to consult Hynd and Cohen (1983), Springer and Deutsch (1984) and Duane (1989). The research, however, is of a highly specialist kind.

We noted above that although the left hemisphere is normally involved in the control of speech, there are some individuals for whom the right hemisphere is involved and that the majority of these are left-handers. This brings us to the issue of 'laterality', under which may be included not only handedness but also eyedness. It is a matter of familiar experience that the majority of people use the right hand for all or most tasks involving fine motor control but that others show varying degrees of left-handedness. In the case of eyedness the majority are known to sight with the right eye in aiming tasks such as rifle shooting, though a significant number are left-eyed.

The relation of all this to dyslexia, however, is far from clear. A large amount of research has been carried out in the attempt to discover whether among poor readers there is an enlarged proportion of left-handers but the results have been bewilderingly contradictory (for sources, see in particular Thomson 1984, p. 79; Annett 1985, pp. 85–7). It is possible that different criteria for handedness have been used by different researchers, but this is quite insufficient to explain the discrepant findings. It should be noted that even when a positive relationship has been found between dyslexia and unusual handedness the differences have seldom been major ones. Thus Geschwind and Behan (1982) report a study of 253 extreme left-handers of whom 24 reported dyslexia or stuttering – scarcely a large proportion, albeit larger than the figure for the extreme right-handers, which was 2. Similarly Naidoo (1972) in her two groups of dyslexic subjects found that 27 per cent and 21 per cent wrote with their left hands, compared with 9 per cent and 10 per cent in her two control groups, while her figures for cross-laterality (that is, right-handedness with left-eyedness or left-handedness with right-eyedness) were 50 per cent and 68 per cent in the case of the dyslexic groups and 41 per cent and 38 per cent in the case of the controls. Even, therefore, if there were no negative findings the use of unusual handedness or cross-laterality as a criterion for dyslexia would still be very unwise.

A particularly interesting contribution to the study of handedness has been made recently by Annett (1985). What she has proposed is a 'right-shift' theory of handedness. According to this theory one should start by considering a situation in which the performance of fine motor skills could be undertaken equally by either hand. It is then postulated that in humans there is a gene which causes a 'shift to the right'. This is to say, in effect, that the presence of this gene causes an individual to be more 'right-handed' than he or she otherwise would have been and also causes the control of all or most speech mechanisms to be sited in the left hemisphere. Those in whom the gene is present are described as 'RS+', those in whom it is absent as 'RS–'. More strictly, if the gene is present on both members of a pair of chromosomes (*alleles*), the notation is 'RS++'; if it is present on one allele but not the other the notation is 'RS+–', while if it is present on neither allele the notation is 'RS––'. It is assumed that RS+ is dominant in that, for instance, left-hemisphere control of speech is likely to be found both in cases of RS++ and cases of RS+–. (Individuals with the same alleles for a particular gene are referred to by geneticists as *homozygotes*, those in whom the alleles are different as *heterozygotes*. The word *genotype* refers to an individual's genetic constitution, the word *phenotype* to the apparent visible or measurable characteristic; and if a characteristic is present in the phenotype when the genotype is heterozygotic, that characteristic is said to be *dominant*.) Annett's hypothesis is that two different factors determine handedness and 'brainedness': the first is the presence or absence of the RS+ gene; the second is the operation of chance factors. If chance factors alone were operating, so she argues, then if one were to compare the performance of the two hands on a particular task, for instance the manipulation of pegs, and calculate the 'difference score' between them, and if one then repeated the same procedure with a large number of subjects the 'difference scores' would form a normal distribution. (For an illustration of this point and a diagram which assumes the absence of the gene in non-humans, see Annett 1985, p. 253.) It is suggested that in humans the observed frequencies of a particular characteristic will be the result of these two factors operating in conjunction. She also hypothesizes that the RS+ gene is stronger in females than in males and stronger in the single-born than in twins.

It is a consequence of the theory that, in the author's words:

> There can be no absolute assertions such as 'all right-handers are...' or 'no left-handers are...'. The task of working out the right-shift theory involves trying to work out just what proportions of so-called right- and left-handers should be left- and right-brained, have right- or left-handed children, or suffer advantages and disadvantages of intellectual growth.
>
> (ibid., p. 260)

In the later part of the book she shows how the theory makes good sense of many of the observed frequencies of such occurrences, for instance the relative rarity in right-handers of right-hemisphere lateralization of speech, the increased incidence of left-handedness in the relatives of left-handers, and so on.

In a later chapter she tentatively suggests, on the basis of findings reported by herself and a colleague (Annett and Kilshaw 1984), that there may be an excess of dyslexics not only among the RS-- but also among the RS++. If this is right it implies that both too much and too little dextrality are risk factors in dyslexia.

Finally, there is research in which post-mortem examinations have been carried out on the brains of a number of individuals with learning difficulties and comparisons made with normal brains. This, too, is a highly technical subject, and we shall limit ourselves to an attempt to highlight what seem to be some of the more important points.

In much of the research the area of the brain chosen for special study was the planum temporale; this is part of the surface of the temporal lobes on each side of the brain. Initial research (Geschwind and Levitsky 1968) had shown that in an unselected autopsy population there was asymmetry between the two plana in 75 per cent of the cases. However, when the brains of those with learning difficulties were examined the plana were invariably symmetrical (Galaburda *et al.* 1987), and this has been found to be true in all eight cases examined to date (Galaburda 1989). In addition all eight brains to a greater or lesser extent showed structural abnormalities, including ectopias (intrusions of cells from one layer to another) and dysplasias (disorganizations of cells within a cell layer).

Galaburda and his colleagues have been cautious in drawing conclusions. It makes sense, however, to suppose that the *balance* between the two halves of the brain is different in dyslexics and that because of the presence of ectopias and dysplasias unusual connections have been formed. If this is right, it would follow that the brain mechanisms available for interaction with the environment are likely to be different. It is in fact widely agreed (though the matter has not been conclusively demonstrated) that dyslexics excel in certain areas – for instance in art, architecture and engineering – and it makes good sense to suppose that there are anatomical reasons for this. (For further discussion of this point see Geschwind 1982, and for a paper entitled 'The advantages of being dyslexic' see Masland 1976.)

In the concluding section (p. 867) of their 1987 paper Galaburda *et al.* write as follows:

> Indirect evidence suggests that asymmetry of the planum results from the greater pruning down of one of the sides during late fetal life and infancy, a process that implicates asymmetry of developmental neuronal loss. Symmetry, on the other hand, reflects failure of asymmetrical cell loss to occur. The exuberant growth of the otherwise smaller side in the symmetrical cases might produce complex qualitative alterations in the functional properties of the system.

Some of their early speculations had been concerned with the role of testosterone. Their suggestion in this paper is that it may have 'a direct effect on the right side in leftward asymmetrical brains and on the left side in rightward asymmetrical brains, probably through interference with the process of neuronal loss that would otherwise lead to asymmetry' (p. 867). In this connection, further evidence has been presented (Tallal and Katz 1989) in support of theories proposing 'hormone-mediated brain development deficits' (p. 193).

Much remains to be discovered. What is clear is that in the case of all eight brains so far studied there have been marked abnormalities; and this finding provides some degree of support for the more general view that the difficulties of the dyslexic are constitutional in origin.

4

The evidence from genetics

Hinshelwood (1917) entitles his third chapter 'Hereditary congenital word-blindness'. He starts by referring to a family of eleven children, of whom the first seven had no literacy problems; thereafter he documents the difficulties of the remaining four, all of whom were boys, along with the difficulties of their nephew and niece, the children of an elder sister who was not herself affected. He is, in effect, making two separate but related claims. The first is that the similarities in clinical presentation between these six cases justify the use of a single diagnostic category (which he calls 'word-blindness'); the second is that the condition is sometimes hereditary. The case for both these claims appears to be strong. With regard to the first, it is plain that, despite differences in nomenclature, others among the early writers, in particular Orton (1937), MacMeeken (1939), Hallgren (1950) and Hermann (1959), were talking about children with basically the same group of difficulties. The second, however, requires further discussion.

On the issue of genetics Critchley (1970) is uncompromising. According to him 'We owe to genetics the most cogent single argument in support of the conception of a constitutional 'specific type of dyslexia among the miscellany of cases of poor readers' (p. 89). Critchley's view is that problems with reading may occur for a variety of reasons but that among poor readers there are some who exhibit 'specific developmental dyslexia' – an identifiable condition, or group of conditions, which needs to be distinguished from poor reading in general.

Now one cannot, of course, legitimately argue for the presence of a hereditary factor solely on the basis of the fact that parent and child both have literacy problems, since social influences could be invoked as an alternative (or even interacting) cause. In the case of the nephew and the niece mentioned by Hinshelwood, however, this explanation seems somewhat far-fetched, since it would have to be assumed that the social factors allegedly leading to illiteracy were operative only in the case of four members of the original family of eleven children and that the unaffected eldest child then re-enacted a pattern of behaviour which she had learned in childhood and which generated literacy problems in her own children. Indeed, even from this kind of evidence on its own it is hard to resist the conclusion that heredity plays some part. In the words of Finucci *et al.* (1976, p. 18), 'very good readers and very poor readers exist side by side in sibships, in contrast to what would be expected if a child were copying the behaviour of older sibs'.

There is, however, a much more powerful technique available, viz. that of studying the differences between monozygotic and dizygotic twins. Many such comparisons have been made, and invariably the concordance rate has been higher in the case of the former, reaching 100% in some of the studies (LaBuda and DeFries 1988). Comparisons using more elaborate statistical techniques have been reported both in the LaBuda and DeFries paper and in papers by DeFries *et al.* (1987) and Stevenson *et al.* (1987). Ideally it would be interesting to carry out tests on monozygotic dyslexic twins who had been reared apart, but this will clearly never be possible on any large scale.

That a hereditary factor plays a part in some cases of dyslexia cannot, therefore, be seriously doubted. What is very much less certain is how exactly such a factor operates.

The first systematic attempt to answer this question was made by Hallgren (1950). His conclusion was that the transmission took place via a dominant gene that was autosomal. (In man there are twenty-two pairs of autosomes, that is, chromosomes not primarily concerned with sex determination, along with the two 'sex chromosomes', XX in the female and XY in the male.) His study was most meticulously carried out, and quite apart from his investigations of heredity there are many other valuable observations made on the basis of detailed neurological, psychological and educational examinations.

Most of the children whom he investigated had attended a

child guidance clinic in Stockholm, though a number of others had been picked out from a secondary school where special provision was made for children with literacy problems. In all, he was able to study 116 dyslexics ('probands' or 'index cases', i.e. those who initially came to the attention of the investigator), along with 160 affected relatives, viz. 96 parents and 64 sibs. Of the 276 studied, 21 were said to be 'borderline' in respect of specific dyslexia.

When pedigree data of this kind are available it is possible to test a variety of hypotheses about the mode of transmission. To take the simplest case first, if a dominant characteristic is transmitted entirely via the Y-chromosome it can never occur in females since all females are XX. Since there are dyslexic females, this possibility in the case of dyslexia is ruled out. Another general principle is this: if a characteristic is entirely transmitted via the X-chromosome, the mating of an affected father with an unaffected mother cannot yield any affected male offspring since male offspring would inherit only the Y-chromosome from the father. In Hallgren's data there were 50 families in which there was mating between an affected father and an unaffected mother and 40 families in which there was mating between an unaffected father and an affected mother. In the first case there were 50 affected sons and 26 affected daughters; in the second case there were 54 affected sons and 20 affected daughters. Since there is no significant difference between these ratios Hallgren concludes that there cannot be transmission via the X-chromosome. Since transmission via the Y-chromosome has already been excluded, the only remaining alternative is autosomal transmission. On the basis of other evidence, in particular the very high frequency with which dyslexia was found in the children of affected parents, he argues that the gene in question must be dominant rather than recessive; hence his overall conclusion is that the mode of transmission is autosomal and dominant.

There are, of course, many methodological difficulties when pedigrees are investigated in this way. For certain calculations one needs to know the numbers of dyslexics in the general population, and it is very difficult to do this with any confidence. Hallgren himself worked on a figure of 10% but admits his calculations have a margin of error. Secondly there are possible uncertainties over diagnosis. In particular, although in the case of children there is relatively little difficulty in carrying out a detailed examination – and it is clear that Hallgren successfully did this on a large scale – to test parents with the same degree of thoroughness is by no means easy. Thirdly, although a particular characteristic, such as dyslexia, may be present in the genotype it may for various reasons fail to manifest itself in the phenotype (see Chapter 3 for an explanation of these terms); and this limits the certainty that can be attached to particular conclusions. In their appraisal of Hallgren's work Finucci *et al.* (1976) write: 'While the size of Hallgren's sample is impressive and his genetic analysis careful, his method of establishing reading disability among adults is questionable, undermining thereby the strength of his conclusions' (p. 3). They themselves studied 20 families and concluded that 'no uniform pattern of transmission is evident; and for any model that might be proposed, there are exceptions'. Even now, however, Hallgren's view has not been decisively ruled out. Thus Stewart (1989) has suggested that the theory of autosomal dominance is correct but that there is lesser penetrance in the female (where 'penetrance' refers to the proportion of phenotypically affected individuals). The criticism of Hallgren by Finucci *et al.* is perhaps less than fair, since there can be good reasons for a clinical diagnosis even when they are hard to specify.

It is possible that where there is dyslexia in the family a gene or genes located on chromosome 15 may be implicated. The evidence for this, however, is of too technical a kind to be discussed here, and those interested should refer to Smith *et al.* (1983) and Lubs *et al.* (1988).

It is in any case almost certainly an oversimplification to suppose that some day researchers will discover something which turns out to be the 'gene for dyslexia'. One possibility is that the action either of a single gene or of several genes in combination may produce effects on the biochemistry of the body and thus create anomalies in the developing brain. In what circumstances, however, these effects may sometimes fail to become operative is unclear.

5

Ocular and oculo-motor approaches

The evidence cited in Chapter 3 suggested that reading and spelling problems might sometimes arise as a result of an imbalance in the processing functions of the two cerebral hemispheres. This, however, does not exclude the possibility that in other individuals – or even in the same individual – there may be faults at the ocular or oculo-motor level. Such faults, if they occurred, would be expected at least to affect reading and possibly to have 'knock on' effects on spelling and other literacy skills. 'Ocular' faults, as such (short sight, astigmatisms, etc.), are outside the scope of this book. What is important from our point of view is that organisms *search* for information (Gibson 1968), and this necessitates correct motor control of the eyes. It is possible, therefore, that there are faults which can usefully be classified as 'oculo-motor': in these cases it is vision which is ultimately affected, but this need not be due to faults in the eyes as such, which, after all, are simply the external and surface parts of a very complex system.

Like those discussed in the previous chapter the problems in this area are of a complex and technical nature, and again no attempt will be made to treat them exhaustively. A number of references will be given, however, which can be consulted by those wishing for more information.

The research will be considered under three heads, viz. (1) studies of eye movements, (2) studies of vergence, and (3) studies in the use of tinted lenses. The latter should perhaps be classified as 'ocular' rather than as 'oculo-motor', but research in this area merits consideration if only because there are many parents of dyslexic children who ask whether tinted lenses are likely to be of help.

1 Studies of eye movements

It is well established that in normal reading the eyes proceed by what is called 'saccadic' movements. That is to say, instead of moving continuously as the person reads across the page they proceed by short leaps, known as 'saccades'. There is then a brief period without movement before the next leap takes place. There have been many studies, for instance Zangwill and Blakemore (1972), which confirm the widely held view that poor readers sometimes display erratic eye movements (for further sources, see Rayner 1986).

Pavlidis (1981), however, went further than this. In his view the eye movements of the dyslexic showed a distinctive pattern which is not to be found in other poor readers or in those for whom the text is too difficult. He also claimed that when non-symbolic stimuli were used – patches of light appearing success-ively in different positions – the dyslexics again had distinctive eye movements. The presence of this pattern could therefore, on his view, be used as an objective method of diagnosis.

Other researchers, however, have reported themselves unable to replicate Pavlidis's findings (for sources, again see Rayner 1986); and it is possible, though not certain, that the conflicting results are due to differences in selection procedure. If Pavlidis is right, it is perhaps not impossible that the same imbalance between the cerebral hemispheres that results in literacy prob-lems could *also* result in difficulty in following the patches of light; this, however, is at present no more than speculation. It would also be interesting if research could be carried out on the possibility of *training* efficient eye movements. A curious – and perhaps uncomfortable – consequence of treating erratic eye movements as the central criterion for dyslexia is that if the eye movements ceased to be erratic one would have to say that the person was no longer dyslexic. This seems at variance with the well-established finding (Rawson 1978) that dyslexic difficulties, though they can be compensated for, continue throughout life.

2 Studies of vergence

Mention was made in Chapter 3 of the subject of eye dominance. One possibility, so it seemed, was that one of the causes of poor reading might be the failure to establish dominance; and it was the concept of 'dominance' which influenced Stein and Fowler in their initial work in this area (see in particular Stein and Fowler 1982). Afterwards, however, the emphasis shifted to 'vergence' (or 'binocular control'), which is the ability to direct both eyes to an identical point in space. Stein (1990) has argued that when one is looking at small targets, such as letters on a printed page, it is important for the eyes to be accurately converged. He points out that if this does not happen, the words may appear to 'jump about', become blurred, or reverse themselves. By adapting a device known as the 'Dunlop test' (the technical details of which need not concern us), Stein and his colleagues were able, for each individual, to establish with a high degree of accuracy whether stable vergence had been achieved. It was then argued that there are some poor readers ('visual dyslexics') whose difficulties are due to unstable vergence. Finally, it was proposed that in suitable cases one of the two eyes should be covered over ('monocular occlusion') for a period of approximately six months, the hypothesis being that improved binocular control would lead to improved reading.

Various studies were carried out to test this hypothesis. In one of these (Stein and Fowler 1985), it was found that in a sample of 148 dyslexic children 101 (68 per cent) showed unstable vergence on the Dunlop test. Of these children, 61 were given occluding spectacles while other children were given placebo plain spectacles. After six months, 31 of the 61 (51 per cent) showed fixed reference, compared with only 10 (24 per cent) of the placebo group, and these 31 showed on average an improvement of 5.6 months of reading age in the 6 months compared with a loss of 0.4 months on the part of the other 30. They also claimed that the children with unfixed reference made more 'visual' than 'auditory' errors (see below for further explanation and discussion). On the basis of these findings and further use of occluding spectacles during the next twelve months they claim that 'monocular occlusion may thus help one sixth of dyslexic children to develop reliable vergence control and thereby to read' (ibid., p. 69).

This conclusion has not, however, been universally accepted.

Thus when Newman *et al.* (1985) used the Dunlop test in a study of 323 8-year-olds they found no difference between good and poor readers in respect of 'unstable ocular dominance' (that is, vergence control). There appears in fact to be a conflict of evidence on this matter which has not yet been resolved. Further criticisms have been made by Wilsher and Taylor (1986). They begin by pointing out that a child who is given the Dunlop test has to respond orally and that a language-disabled child may make inappropriate responses not because of failure to establish vergence but because of his inability to name the direction of movement correctly. They then argue as follows:

> The researchers displayed their results by comparing reading scores for the group of occluded dyslexics whose Dunlop test score improved, with the group of non-occluded dyslexics whose score did not improve.... It is quite possible that children who *learn* to perform better on the verbal/visual/verbal task of the Dunlop test will be the ones who *learn* to read better. Consequently, selecting the better learners in one group and comparing them with the poor learners in the other group must always produce a significant difference.
>
> (Wilsher and Taylor 1986, pp. 292–3)

Criticisms of the work of Stein and Fowler have also been made by Bishop (1989). Some of the more important of these are as follows:

(a) Even if there is a relationship between unstable vergence and poor reading (which is not, on her view, conclusively established, see above), it would not follow that the relationship is a causal one. Indeed, if it were, one would expect *all* those with unstable vergence to be poor readers, and this is agreed not to be the case.

(b) Stein and Fowler claimed that children with unstable vergence made more 'visual' than 'phonemic' errors. 'Visual errors were: losing the place on the page ...; having to point with a finger to keep the place ...; and missequencing, reversing, and rotating words and letters when reading and writing – e.g. was/saw, no/on, b/d.... Phonemic (auditory) errors consisted of the failure to find rhymes or alliterations for ten common words' (Stein and Fowler 1985, p. 71). However, as Bishop (1989, p. 211) has pointed out: 'the behaviours regarded as evidence of visually based reading problems are open to other interpretations'. This is a matter to which we shall be returning in Chapter 7.

(c) After statistical re-analysis of the data provided by Stein and Fowler [she found that there had been computational errors in their 1985 paper] and appropriate comparison of the various groups (fixed/unfixed reference eye, occlusion/no occlusion, occlusion after six months, etc.), she claims that alternative explanations of the figures have not been ruled out. Thus she agrees that there is a significant relationship between development of stable reference and improvement in reading, but argues that this could be explained in terms of differences in initial reading ability. 'There is no evidence that monocular occlusion in children with unfixed reference results in improved reading scores' (Bishop 1989, p. 214).

It is to the credit of Stein and his colleagues that they were entirely willing to submit their data to independent scrutiny and possible falsification, since, sadly, not all scientists are so open-minded! Stein has in fact offered a reply to Bishop's criticisms and says that further results will be published 'confirming that assisting children to develop good binocular control often helps them to learn to read' (Stein 1989, p. 320).

He is not, of course, disputing that many poor readers have phonological problems (compare Chapter 9 of this book). In the paper cited above (Stein 1990) he suggests that in some individuals vergence problems may coexist with phonological problems, and he has also suggested (personal communication to the authors) that there may be varying degrees of each, from none at all of the one to none at all of the other. Clearly it is an area where the reader needs to keep an open mind until further evidence is forthcoming.

3 Studies in the use of tinted lenses

The starting-point for these investigations appears to have been a paper by Helen Irlen which was delivered to the American Psychological Association in 1983. Mention of this paper is made by Robinson and Miles (1987) – no relation to the present authors – and by Whiting (1988). According to the latter, Irlen claims to have identified a group of symptoms which she refers to as 'scotopic sensitivity syndrome'.

The syndrome was said to include six areas of difficulty: photo-

Check For Spelling mistakes !

phobia, eye strain, poor visual resolution, reduced span of fixation (focus), poor sustained focus and impaired depth perception.... Irlen experimented with using coloured filters to modify the light spectrum available to these clients, and discovered that the use of individually tinted lenses considerably reduced the symptoms or eliminated them altogether, making the reading task relaxing and easy rather than stressful and difficult.

(Whiting 1988, p. 13)

To test this claim Whiting sent out a survey form to 343 individuals who had worn Irlen lenses for twelve months. Of the 155 who replied, many of them reported 'large improvements' in certain areas; for example, 43.9 per cent reported less eye-strain, 37.8 per cent a lesser tendency to skip lines, and 35.5 per cent improved concentration. Some even reported an improvement in handwriting (12.2 per cent) and an improvement in spelling (10.4 per cent). Obviously a survey form asking for opinions is not the ideal research tool, and in a review of the use of colour as a means of helping those with a learning disability Howell and Stanley (1988) conclude that 'research to separate mood and motivational effects from visual effects is recommended' (p. 66). However, O'Connor and Sofo (1988) claim that 'Helen Irlen's work was a major breakthrough' (p. 12), and positive claims (albeit more cautious ones) are made by Cheetham and Ovenden (1987). In contrast, Winter (1987) has reported a study which 'provides no evidence to suggest that Irlen lenses improve visual performance'.

It would appear, therefore, that in the case of tinted lenses, just as in the case of monocular occlusion, the published evidence is contradictory. It could perhaps be argued that the majority of studies lend support to the view that tinted lenses can sometimes make reading easier. It would be agreed on all sides, however, that, if this is so, more research is needed in order to determine why these results occur and to separate out the possible influence of Hawthorne or placebo effects. It would also be interesting to know whether some normal readers can also be helped.

Finally, as a caution, we should like to quote from an article by the mother of a reading-disabled boy (Peterson 1987):

For nine years I have watched helplessly as Scot struggles with schoolwork.... His vision definitely appeared to improve with the use of some coloured overlays or lenses. However... after an initial burst of enthusiastic use, Scot's glasses have gradually fallen into disuse and lie forgotten in a corner of his school bag along with the odd banana skin and torn out pages of a book.

Advocates of tinted lenses have never claimed that *all* children can be helped by their use, nor has any such claim been made for the occlusion techniques mentioned under (2) above. Sadly, however, there is risk when any new line of research receives publicity that the unwary will expect too much from it.

In addition, those who recommend either occlusion or tinted glasses need to take into account the possible social consequences of their use. For instance, it is worth asking whether the child will be teased by her classmates because of her unusual spectacles, whether she will be scolded if she forgets to wear them, and whether the issue may lead to disputes within the family. These are complications which can sometimes be overlooked. Where a form of treatment is known for certain to be effective the risk of such 'side-effects' may well seem acceptable, but where there is doubt the decision is more difficult. One of the most serious dangers is that of disappointment; and it is particularly sad if high hopes are raised, only to be dashed when the treatment proves ineffective. This is something about which enquirers should always be warned.

6

Clinical and experimental studies

The previous chapters have shown that, according to a number of investigators, including in particular Morgan, Hinshelwood, Orton, MacMeeken, Hallgren and Critchley, it is possible to identify a group of individuals whose literacy difficulties make them distinctive. On their view there is a homogeneity among members of this group which justifies use of the same diagnostic label, whether 'word blindness', 'strephosymbolia', 'dyslexia', or some other. Although, as was pointed out in the Preface, different labels carry different theoretical implications, it is plain that the above writers were all describing similar individuals. The aim of the present chapter is to try to indicate what have been found to be the distinctive characteristics of those who can be classified as 'dyslexic' in this standard sense.

One of the best ways of starting to learn about dyslexia is to meet dyslexic individuals and their families and simply listen to what they have to say, and this is a policy which we recommend to readers. It is also helpful to study the literature on individual cases. There are two full-scale autobiographies written by dyslexics, those by Simpson (1980) and Hampshire (1981). Briefer autobiographical sketches have also been written by Mautner (1984), Martin (1986), Batty (1986) and N.L. Stein (1987). In addition many descriptions have been provided by people other than the dyslexics themselves, sometimes, though not always, as a lead-in to more generalized conclusions about research or teaching (see, for instance, Hinshelwood 1917;

Gillingham and Stillman 1969; Naidoo 1972; Rawson 1978; Miles 1983, 1987; Thomson 1984; Snowling 1987).

Attempts have also been made to identify dyslexia in distinguished individuals of earlier generations. Some of these attempts, regrettably, are based on rather scanty evidence, although a notable exception is the paper by Aaron *et al.* (1988), in which there are detailed biographical studies of Thomas Alva Edison, Woodrow Wilson, Hans Christian Andersen and Leonardo da Vinci. In these four cases the cumulative evidence for dyslexia is extremely convincing. We are told, for instance, that Andersen 'never learned to spell properly' and that a contemporary critic asked, 'When will such a prolific writer... learn to write his mother tongue correctly?' (this despite corrections made to his manuscripts by his friend, Edvard Collin). In his diary Hans Andersen wrote: 'If only I could show some progress but I'm scared of the exam, I'm balancing somewhere between the two bottom marks.' In a letter to Edvard Collin he wrote of 'something restless and hasty in my soul which makes it twice as difficult for me to get to grips with languages' (Aaron *et al.* 1988, p. 532). Many will remember Hans Andersen's delightful story, *The Ugly Duckling*, in which a bird who was a total 'misfit' among the ducks turns out afterwards to be a beautiful swan – an allegory which should certainly be taken to heart by struggling dyslexics!

Despite the differences between individuals there is clearly a common pattern. A characteristic which virtually all dyslexics share (and which can therefore be accepted as a definitional characteristic) is the contrast between their skills in certain areas and their incongruous weakness in others. It follows, of course, that one of the most important signs to look for clinically is that of discrepancy. We shall be discussing later the question of the use of intelligence tests with dyslexics. For the present it is important to note that children who score highly on such tests – or, in traditional but somewhat questionable terminology, have a 'high IQ' – can sometimes be very weak at reading and spelling; and it follows that the results of intelligence tests, if suitably interpreted, can supply important evidence that in certain areas the child may have considerable strengths. This is also true of adults; and Miles (1983, 1987) has noted how those dyslexics aiming to go to college or university often obtained high scores on the Advanced Raven Matrices Test (Raven 1965). Not all 'underachievers' (that is, those whose performance on reading and spelling tests is lower than might have been predicted from their intelligence level) are necessarily dyslexic (compare Chapter 12); but underachievement is at least an important pointer.

Another common characteristic shared by many dyslexics whose cases have been described is lack of success at school, at least in the early stages. Thus Batty (1986) tells us: 'When I entered my secondary school I was automatically put in the bottom class ... I could hardly read and could hardly write.' Then, at a later stage, 'I was put in for most of the CSEs, which I didn't work for, one reason being that I was told I was so stupid anyhow that I wouldn't get any qualifications' (p. 124). Martin (1986) writes: 'Even after I was confirmed dyslexic, little changed at school and some teachers still considered me lazy and that I now used dyslexia as an excuse ... I was the only student to fail General Studies; this I attribute largely to not reading books or newspapers as I found reading difficult and always lost interest' (pp. 119–20). Many dyslexics are able to laugh about their misfortunes, as can be seen from the following passage in Hampshire (1981, p. 11): 'A "bad day" for me is a day when I have spent hours carefully embroidering "passionetly lovd" instead of "passionately loved" on a corner of my husband's handkerchief.' Yet there may still be uncertainty and even bitterness, as is shown in the following words by Mautner (1984, p 309): 'More importantly, education and success have not eliminated the strong emotional reactions of frustration, embarrassment, and anger that are a result of my life with dyslexia'. Usually some proficiency in reading is achieved even though spelling in most cases remains weak. In many cases dyslexics have achieved success; and it is the considered opinion of Rawson, one of the leading American authorities on the subject, that in general 'advice to keep the educational and occupational sights very modest would have been inappropriate' (Rawson 1978, p. 82). Wise suggestions from the parent of a dyslexic will be found in Hartwig (1984); for example he encourages parents to be patient but not to be overprotective or do things for the child which he can do for himself.

Starting with the assumption that an identifiable 'syndrome' or 'pattern of difficulties' is to be found, Miles (1983, 1987) has made various attempts to specify what a 'typical' dyslexic would be like. He does not claim that all the signs which he describes will co-occur in any one individual, and he agrees that the same signs will sometimes be found in non-dyslexics, albeit less frequently.

What he continually found was that the children and adults whom he assessed had difficulties in certain distinctive areas, which may be summarized as follows: uncertainty over left and right, becoming 'tied up' in trying to say or repeat long words, difficulty in carrying out certain apparently easy subtraction tasks, difficulty in learning arithmetical tables, and difficulty in saying the months of the year, particularly if the task was to say them in reverse order. He also noticed a tendency to confuse 'b' and 'd' at an age when most children might have been expected to have grown out of this. Like others before him he noticed that the difficulties frequently seemed to run in families and that they were more common in boys than in girls. He believed that the 'recall of digits' items which occur in traditional intelligence tests such as the Stanford–Binet (Terman and Merrill 1960) and the WISC (Wechsler 1976) were misplaced as measures of intelligence and that a weak performance on these items could be regarded as a diagnostic indicator of dyslexia. Basically, Miles's argument was that incongruous weakness in any one of these areas would be of no particular significance, since incongruous events do indeed occur from time to time, and a person might 'just happen' to be weak at, say, recall of digits for no particular reason. Indeed, even if a second improbable response was noted, for example if the person showed uncertainty over the months of the year, this might still be 'accidental', since there would be nothing 'special' in the fact that two improbable events were found in the same person. If, however, the same pattern regularly showed itself, with three, four, five or more 'incongruous' signs being present, and if similar signs were also found to be present in one or more members of the same family, it would become progressively more uncomfortable, so he argues, to regard these signs as coincidental or without significance.

Clinical observations, however, for all their importance at the start of an inquiry, are of limited value since they cannot on their own lead to valid generalization. Thus one does not always know by what criteria a particular individual was diagnosed as dyslexic, and even if the criteria are specified one does not know how frequently the allegedly 'dyslexic signs' would be expected to occur among other individuals, whether dyslexic or not. Nor is it possible without systematic research to say with certainty that this or that response *is* a dyslexic sign; indeed, an interesting example in this connection is that of unusual handedness: many reports on dyslexics call attention to the existence of unusual handedness in a way which implies that this is one of the reasons for the diagnosis (for instance, Gillingham and Stillman 1969). In view of the diverse findings in the literature, however (for sources see Chapter 3), it is far from clear that this procedure is legitimate. In the case of any sign which is a possible candidate for being an indicator of dyslexia experienced clinicians may say, 'This *feels like* a dyslexic response', and they may regularly be right; but unless they are prepared to specify the criteria which they are using they are in effect relying on personal mystique, with the result that communication with others is not possible. If there is to be significant advance mystique needs to be replaced by science.

Now when people make what is called a 'clinical diagnosis', what is happening from the scientific point of view is that they are making use of certain signs – small ones, perhaps, and varying from one individual to another – but signs which are in principle capable of being specified. Such a specification was attempted by Miles (1982). The items mentioned above (difficulty over left–right, etc.), which he believed on the basis of clinical experience to be indicative of dyslexia, were brought together into a test, and standard instructions for administration were provided. Incorrect answers (and various other responses, see below) were scored as 'plus', that is, 'dyslexia positive'; correct answers were scored as 'minus' ('dyslexia negative'), while an intermediate category ('zero') was used if the responses were neither unambiguously 'plus' nor unambiguously 'minus'. One way in which the clinical 'feel' of the case could be taken into account was that the outcome (plus, zero, or minus) did not simply depend on the *correctness* of the response: the result could also be scored as positive if, for instance, the subject repeated the question under his breath, hesitated, or seemed to be using some special compensatory strategy. Miles emphasizes the need to make a diagnosis on the basis of the total picture. Typically, in his view, a dyslexic is one who, despite adequate intelligence, has at least a *history* of reading difficulty, is a poor speller, and comes out as 'positive' on a significant number of items from the Bangor Dyslexia Test. He does not regard it as necessary to specify what exactly constitutes 'adequate' intelligence or what should constitute a 'significant' number of positive indicators, since this may vary from one individual to the next. Nor does he claim that the items in the Bangor Dyslexia Test are the only possible criteria; indeed any task which reliably distinguishes dyslexics from non-dyslexics could be included in a diagnostic battery. The items in question were chosen both for convenience of administration and as a representative selection designed to give test users the 'feel' of what a typical dyslexic is like. An investigator might well discover that a particular individual had problems with 'east' and 'west' or with 'port' and 'starboard', and this would be as much a 'positive indicator' as uncertainty over 'left' and 'right'.

If there is evidence of lack of intelligence or lack of opportunity the diagnosis will, of course, be more problematic; and if the child is aged less than 7, various changes can be made in the diagnostic procedure; thus a younger child could be asked to say the days of the week in place of the months of the year or perhaps be given tasks involving segmentation or rhyming (compare Chapter 9).

While it is possible that a positive diagnosis of dyslexia may be indicative of anomalies at the neurological level (see Chapter 3), the educational significance of such a diagnosis is that other dyslexic signs may be expected. A diagnosis of dyslexia is therefore in an important sense a 'bet' (Miles 1983, p. 23) and can be shown to be correct or incorrect according to what the person does on other occasions. If the diagnosis is positive then steps can immediately be taken to forestall future difficulties and the appropriate teaching programme (see Chapter 10) can be arranged. In addition, even though the precise nature of the neurological anomalies is not yet known, it is possible to reassure the child or adult that he is no more to be blamed for his problems than someone who is deaf or lame, since they have arisen from the way in which he is made. It is also worth while reminding dyslexics that in so-called 'right hemisphere' tasks (see Chapter 3) they may well have exceptional talent. Miles also reports that he has found it useful to explain the results in detail to the child and his parents and to check with them whether the diagnosis seemed to them to 'make sense' (see Miles 1988). He has also indicated that opportunities can be made to discuss with both children and adults the frustrations which they have felt or the teasing which some of them may be experiencing (or have experienced) at school as a result of their difficulties.

Once the specification has been made as to which responses count as 'plus', 'zero' and 'minus', a check on the validity of the items in the Bangor Dyslexia Test immediately becomes possible – not, indeed, a proof that they are genuinely indicators of dyslexia (since one would then have to specify other criteria for dyslexia as a yardstick!) – but as a way of showing the counter-hypothesis to be mistaken. One way of refuting the 'dyslexia-indicator' hypothesis would be to show that 'dyslexia positive' results on these items are as frequent in non-dyslexics as in dyslexics. Miles made a comparison between 132 dyslexics, aged 7 and upwards, and 132 controls (adequate spellers) matched as far as possible for age and intelligence level in respect of seven of the ten items on the Bangor Dyslexia Test. The following table has been extracted from Miles (1983, p. 56). It relates to 160 of these children, viz. those between the ages of 9 years 0 months and 12 years 11 months (80 dyslexics and 80 controls), and it shows what percentage of each came out as 'dyslexia positive' on the different items.

	Dyslexics	Controls
Digits reversed	80	48
Left-right	78	42
Polysyllables	56	24
Subtraction	58	19
Tables	96	51
Months forwards	60	13
Months reversed	86	28

This table confirms that the dyslexics obtained more 'pluses' than the controls in all seven items. Had they not done so, the whole basis for the Bangor Dyslexia Test would have been called in question.

Various other points about this table are worth mention. In the first place, no one item on its own is sufficient to provide a firm diagnosis either way. The fact that only 13 per cent of the controls came out as 'positive' on 'months forwards' means that difficulty with this item is a strong positive indicator, but success on it is relatively uninformative since even in the case of the dyslexics 40 per cent had no difficulty. Conversely, the fact that 96 per cent of the dyslexics came out as 'positive' on the tables item means that a 'minus' on this item is a strong counter-indicator of dyslexia, whereas a 'plus' is relatively uninformative since 51 per cent of the controls came out as 'positive'. It is the combination of results on which the diagnosis has to be made. Secondly, it is a mistake to suppose that dyslexics will invariably show a particular difficulty and that non-dyslexics will never do so. The position is rather that in certain areas dyslexics are more at risk. This, indeed, is in no way surprising, since there is very little that dyslexics cannot be taught if they put in sufficient time and effort; it is rather that there are certain things which they do not pick up easily. Conversely, those who are not dyslexic may 'miss out' on certain skills not because of any developmental anomaly but simply through lack of the requisite experience. Further use has been made of the Bangor Dyslexia Test in a large-scale survey. This survey involved all children born in England, Wales and Scotland during a particular week in April 1970. Data were collected of many different kinds, both at the time of birth and in 1975 and 1980. On this last occasion it was possible to include tests of single-word reading, of spelling and of intelligence – the Similarities and Matrices items from the British Ability Scales (Elliott *et al.* 1983) – along with the 'left-right', 'months forwards' and 'months reversed' items from the Bangor Dyslexia Test and the Recall of Digits item from the British Ability Scales, a basically similar item to that in the Bangor Dyslexia Test but involving only 'digits forwards'. The results are reported in a paper by Miles and Haslum (1986). Those whose reading or spelling was below expectation as judged by their performance on the 'intelligence' items were classed as 'under-achievers', and a further subdivision was made between those underachievers who produced a specified number of 'positive indicators' on the 'left–right', 'months forwards', 'months reversed' and 'digit span' items and those who did not. The boy : girl ratio was found to be far higher among the dyslexic under-achievers than among the non-dyslexic underachievers; and various other predictions were made which would have been falsified if those picked out as 'dyslexic' had behaved no differently from other children in the survey. The authors indicate that they regard the dyslexia concept as of value only if it implies some kind of anomaly of development, and they claim from their figures that when 'anomalous' (i.e. dyslexic) children are picked out by the criteria which they specify (derived from the Bangor Dyslexia Test), the anomaly hypothesis has 'resisted refutation'. (For further evidence on the boy : girl ratio in dyslexics see Finucci and Childs 1981.)

Mention was made earlier of the fact that dyslexics sometimes obtain high scores on certain items in traditional intelligence tests. This is an area, however, where clinical observation needs to be supplemented by systematic comparison. A large amount of evidence is available on the performance of poor readers on the various sub-tests of the WISC and WISC-R (Wechsler 1976).

Details of these sub-tests will not be given here, except for four of them. These are

1　the Arithmetic sub-test, which involves a set of arithmetical items of graded difficulty,
2　the Coding sub-test, in which the child is shown ten simple patterns (for instance a line with a dot over it), each paired with a digit; then, when digits are presented on their own with a 'box' underneath, the task is to fill the 'box' with the correct pattern,
3　the Information sub-test, which is basically a test of general knowledge, and
4　the Digit Span sub-test, in which the child has to repeat strings of auditorily presented digits in forwards order and further strings in reverse order.

The main finding is that poor readers regularly tend to be weaker at these four sub-tests than at any of the others. This is a finding which has held up over many different investigations (for detailed evidence see Rugel 1974, pp. 51–3, and Spache 1976, p. 140, and for a theoretical discussion Miles and Ellis 1981). In the case of a dyslexic child, therefore, it is very unwise to cite an IQ figure (whether 'verbal', 'performance', or 'full-scale') without qualification, since the addition of scores representing a child's strengths to scores representing his weaknesses is unlikely to yield any very useful measure. Similarly Thomson (1982) has compared dyslexics and non-dyslexics on a variety of items from the 1979 version of the British Ability Scales (Elliott *et al.* 1983); and here, too, it was found that the dyslexics showed a distinctive pattern in comparison with the controls – weakness at recall of digits, at arithmetic, at certain types of visual recall, and at a task described as 'speed of information processing', where the child has, for instance, to place a ring round the highest of a series of five numbers. These differences held up in the case of children at three different age levels (8 to 10 years, 11 to 13 years, and 14 to 16 years).

It does not follow from these results that intelligence tests should never be used with dyslexics; on the contrary many of the items provide them with an opportunity to show their distinctive skills. It is wise policy, however, to examine the sub-test scores individually and to treat the overall score with caution; otherwise there is a danger that one may underestimate their ability in some areas just because they are weak in others.

A difficulty which is often reported at clinical assessments is slowness at copying from the blackboard. There is no reason to doubt such reports, but the issue is clearly one which admits of systematic research, since there are many ways in which the 'blackboard' situation can be replicated in the laboratory. In particular it is possible to measure the time needed for the reading of visual displays.

Evidence suggesting that dyslexics are slow at this task has been reported by Ellis and Miles (1977). When arrays of 4, 5, 6 and 7 digits were flashed on a screen it was found that dyslexics (average age 12 years) needed more time to produce the correct response than controls (average age 8 years) matched for spelling age. In another experiment, this time with adult dyslexics (university and college students), Miles (1986) required his subjects to compare a written sentence with a diagram, both of them presented on a monitor screen, and to indicate whether the sentence was true or false by pressing one or other of two keys. For example, one of the stimuli was:

b   d

The b is to the right of the d

where the 'false' key had to be pressed. For this particular item the dyslexics required on average about 5 seconds to respond correctly, compared with just over 2 seconds for the controls; and there were still differences between the two groups, though less marked ones, when the 'up–down' dimension was used instead of the 'left-right' dimension and the stimuli were a 'star' (*) and a 'plus' (+) as opposed to a 'b' and a 'd'. These results suggest not only that dyslexics are slow at information processing in childhood but that they remain so into adult life. In the same paper Miles (1986) reports the case of a dyslexic student who, despite daily practice over a full month, made only very modest gains in his ability to respond quickly to arrays of five visually presented digits, being in fact slower than a non-dyslexic student who had just started to learn Russian and who put in the same amount of practice with Russian characters.

It may also be helpful to consider a set of experiments carried out by Tallal and Piercy (1973) in which children who had been diagnosed as aphasic (having obtained very low scores on tests of receptive and/or expressive language) were found to be slow at processing auditory stimuli (bleeps) but not visual stimuli (light flashes). In one experiment, with children aged between 6 years 3 months and 9 years 3 months, the stimulus comprised two tones, one high and one low, whose duration varied between 75 and 250 milliseconds (ms, that is thousandths of a second), and which were presented at inter-stimulus intervals (ISIs) of between 8 and 305 ms. At the start of the experiment a training procedure was carried out, using a tone which lasted for 75 ms. Initially the subjects were rewarded for pressing the correct panel, from a choice of two, according to whether the high or low tone had sounded. Thereafter they were trained to respond to each of the four possible two-element stimulus patterns (high-high, high-low, low-high, low-low) by pressing the panels accordingly (right-right, right-left, left-right, left-left). All the subjects learned to respond correctly. When training was complete the experimenters systematically varied the tone duration and the ISI. They found that when the tone duration was 250 ms there was no difference between the aphasics and the controls, regardless of ISI. If the tone duration was 125 ms, however, then for ISIs of 150 ms or less the aphasics made more errors, while if the ISI was very brief (15 ms) they made more errors even when the time duration was raised to 175 ms. These results suggest that developmental aphasics cannot deal with auditory information at the normal rate.

When Tallal (1980) used the same procedure with poor readers she found that they made no errors when the ISIs were 500 ms, but that at shorter ISIs they made many more errors than the controls. She also found a high correlation between the number of errors made by her subjects on this test and the number of errors made when they were required to read nonsense words. Since not all her poor readers had difficulty with these two tasks she suggests that difficulty in rapid auditory perception may be more specifically related to language deficits than to reading deficits as such. How far the subjects in these experiments were able to verbalize what was required and how far, if at all, they were helped by doing so cannot be known for certain. What is plain is that when poor readers are slow at dealing with incoming information this is not limited to visual information. More speculatively, it is arguable from these experiments that developmental dyslexia is a milder variant of developmental aphasia: thus although receptive language is adequate in dyslexia and expressive language not markedly affected, at least on standard tests, the two conditions are alike in that in both cases speed of information processing is affected.

Another area where clinical impressions have been supplemented by systematic research is that of mathematics. There is no doubt that it is *possible* to be dyslexic and yet be a very successful mathematician: this is shown conclusively in a paper by Jansons (1987) who describes his personal experiences as a dyslexic. In addition Joffe (1983) has reported that 10 per cent of her dyslexic subjects 'excelled' in the subject. Yet many dyslexics appear to have difficulties; and the most likely conclusion seems to be that, although success is possible, there are *certain areas* of mathematics which present difficulty. This, at least, is the conclusion which follows from a carefully conducted piece of research by Steeves (1983).

Steeves begins by describing an episode which took place among some 9-year-olds at a school for dyslexics:

> A small group of boys were preparing to make a three-dimensional model. Some engineering graph paper was being distributed to a group of six boys, and before the teacher had reached the sixth boy, an interval of no more than twelve seconds, the first boy called out excitedly that there were 28,000 little squares on his sheet of paper.
>
> (p. 141)

Yet this boy was two years below grade level at both reading and spelling and had come out as only *average* on an arithmetic test. This was an incongruity which Steeves decided to investigate further. She believed that some dyslexics 'exhibited a potential for mathematical talent while at the same time exhibiting a lack of computational efficiency' (p. 144), and she decided to test whether this lack could in part be due to memory deficits.

Her subjects were children aged between 10 and 14 years. She divided them into four groups; (i) 'dyslexics high' (DH), that is, dyslexics with a high score on the Raven Standard Progressive Matrices test (SPM) (Raven 1938), (ii) 'dyslexics average' (DA), that is dyslexics with an average score on the SPM, (iii) non-dyslexics in an advanced (or 'high') class for mathematics (NH), and (iv) non-dyslexics in an average class for mathematics (NA). There were 27 children in each group, and care was taken to ensure suitable matching on age, sex, and type of school. Groups (iii) and (iv) were then given the SPM, and all children were given a mathematics computation test and the Wechsler Memory Test (which includes items such as associate learning and immediate memory span). Some of the main findings were: the NH and DH groups were level on SPM score; the DH scored lower than the NH on the computation test but were level with the NA group, while on the Wechsler Memory Test the DH group scored lower than both the NH and the NA groups. The DA group scored lower than the others throughout.

Steeves concludes that there can be dyslexics with high reasoning power (and hence high mathematical potential) who nevertheless score only at average level on tests of computation, and that their memory skills are inferior to those of non-dyslexics with lower reasoning power.

Similar uneven performances have been reported by Miles (1983, p. 120; 1987, p. 117). For example, there is a very complex mathematical item set at the top grade of 'Superior Adult' in the Terman–Merrill intelligence test (Terman and Merrill 1960); in it the subject is given the height of a tree at the time of planting and at yearly intervals for the next three years. There have been many dyslexic subjects who have grasped the complicated nature of the progressions involved (which can be either arithmetical or geometrical) but have had great difficulty in carrying out what to others would be 'easy' calculations in order to find the right answer, for instance that 27–18 is 9. Miles has also noted that subjects whom he believed to be dyslexic often tended to use their fingers or marks on paper as an aid to calculation, some of them using special strategies, for example going to the nearest multiple of ten and then counting in ones. In addition he found that almost all of them reported difficulty in learning multiplication tables, and if asked to recite, say, the 6-times, 7-times, or 8-times they might 'lose the place', break into the 'wrong' table, or say 'eight eighties' instead of 'eight eights'.

On the basis of experiments with boys aged 12 to 16 Pritchard *et al.* (1989) have argued that dyslexics have fewer 'number facts' available to them than non-dyslexics, where a person is said to 'possess a number fact' if he can give the answer to a sum immediately (for example, 'What is 8×7?') without having to work anything out. They argue that the dyslexic learns to make use of regularities in the number system – and hence, for instance, has no difficulty with the 10-times table – and that the need to use fingers or marks on paper arises because, even if no other regularities are available, he can at least make use of the fact that numbers go up in ones!

If all this evidence is taken in conjunction, there is a good case for believing that the difficulties experienced by dyslexics in mathematics are part and parcel of their other difficulties: it is possible for a dyslexic to be very strong intellectually and yet have distinctive weakness in committing symbolic material to memory, including the symbols of mathematics. One might also expect difficulties over words that are used in mathematics in a distinctive sense, for instance the word 'make' when it is said that 'two and two make four' or the word 'dividend' which in many quarters implies something which people win on the pools! There is no need, incidentally, on the basis of these findings to postulate a special condition, 'dyscalculia', which may or may not accompany dyslexia. It seems rather that the same difficulties which affect reading and spelling may also affect some aspects of calculation. It is not that some dyslexics have difficulty with mathematics and some do not; it is that all of them have difficulty with certain aspects of mathematics – difficulties which many of them, to varying degrees, may learn to overcome.

Relatively little research has been carried out on whether dyslexics have any distinctive personality characteristics. Observers often report, however, that they have come across many dyslexics who seem reluctant to 'commit themselves'; and it is commonly supposed that repeated reproofs ('You are lazy', 'Try harder', etc.) have made them unduly cautious. One systematic study in this area should perhaps be mentioned briefly, viz. that in which Williams and Miles (1985) carried out some explorations with the Rorschach ink-blot test. Information about this test will be found in Klopfer and Kelley (1943). It involves presenting the subjects with ten cards containing various shapes – not representing immediately identifiable objects but capable of being seen in different ways. There is a considerable literature relating certain types of response to certain personality characteristics. Now when they gave this test to dyslexic and non-dyslexic children between the ages of 8 and 16 years, Williams and Miles found that there was nothing wrong with the dyslexics' perception as such (as there is, for instance, in certain types of mental illness), but that they tended, unlike the controls, to restrict themselves to one response per card and not to exploit the many possibilities of the blots – their colour, their detail and what they might look like if turned upside down. Some of the testing was done in North Wales and some in the area of New York; and there were consistent differences between the dyslexics and controls regardless of the venue. The authors suggest that their results provide support for the hypothesis (hitherto based only on informal observation) that dyslexics are reluctant to commit themselves too far because of uncertainty about the consequences. In the light of more recent findings (see Chapter 9) it is possible that their small number of responses may also have been influenced by the amount of effort needed in spontaneously generating words as opposed to responding to words produced by someone else. However that may be, in this particular piece of research the differences between the dyslexics and the controls were extremely clear.

A field of study which has recently attracted attention is that of dyslexia and music. No systematic research has yet been completed; but a booklet (Smith 1988) is available which has collated evidence from various sources and set out a list of some of the main ways in which dyslexics have reported that they find music difficult. The list is a long one; it includes, for instance, reading from a score where there is more than one line of music, coping with repeat marks and with DS and DC signs, remembering a melodic or rhythmic phrase and singing or clapping it back, working out 'left' and 'right' at the keyboard, and transposing from one clef to another. Hubicki (1990) has called attention to the confusion which may be caused by some of the terms used in music, such as 'treble', 'note' and 'key', which in a musical context do not carry their familiar meanings (compare what was said above about 'make' and 'dividend'). On her view it is possible to learn music in a 'multisensory' way, since the pupil needs to learn relationships between the pitch and duration of a sound, the position of the hands on a musical instrument if this sound is to be produced, and the visually presented notation on a musical score.

In general, music seems to be in a similar position to mathematics; that is to say, there is every reason for supposing that a suitably talented dyslexic can succeed at either; in both cases, however, there are basic problems which need to be overcome – not problems of mathematics or music as such but problems of mastering the notation in which mathematical or musical ideas are expressed.

7

The question of sub-types I

One of the commonest of distinctions made in connection with
sub-typing is that between 'visual' and 'auditory' dyslexics. This
distinction originates with Johnson and Myklebust (1967). They
first point out (p. 17) that a deficit can be either verbal or non-
verbal. They then go on to discuss, in the area of verbal
behaviour, the processes involved in speaking and listening and
in reading and writing. 'It is apparent', they say, 'that deficiencies
might be auditory and/or visual in nature' (p. 20).

Despite this reference to 'auditory' and 'visual' problems it is
clear that in the case of dyslexia the authors believe that they are
talking about deficiencies in verbal behaviour. They agree that
there are also some visual learning disabilities which 'affect
nonverbal functions', while others 'interfere with several forms
of symbolic behavior including arithmetic and music' (p. 152).
They take it as self-evident, however, that reading is a verbal
function, and it is within the framework of this assumption that
their distinction between 'auditory dyslexics' and 'visual dyslexics'
is made.

The distinction is expressed as follows:

> The child learns the spoken word and what the letters look like,
> but he cannot associate these images with the way they sound (an
> auditory type of dyslexia). The reverse also can occur. He learns
> what letters sound like but cannot make the normal association
> between these auditory images and their appearance (a visual type
> of dyslexia).
>
> (p. 28)

The authors' use of the word 'image' might well be called in question nowadays, and the importance which they attach to 'intersensory integration' could also be called in question (for evidence, see Vellutino 1979). What is important is the educational practice which they advocate on the basis of the distinction.

Children with auditory involvements respond best to a whole word or ideo-visual approach *during the initial stages of reading instruction.* Because of their problems in auditory perception, memory, and integration, they are unable to handle the skills required for phonetic analysis; in fact some may be able to develop auditory skills *only after having learned a sight vocabulary.* As with the visual dyslexic, however, debilitated functions cannot be ignored. Even though able to learn by a global method, he cannot possibly retain visual images for every word; therefore he must acquire a systematic means of attacking unfamiliar words (our italics).

(pp. 175-6)

There is no doubt, in view of this passage, that they envisage the 'auditory dyslexic' as eventually acquiring auditory skills.

Thus they do not at all see the methods of teaching the two types of dyslexics as mutually exclusive, but only as alternative approaches at the start. They appreciate that it is possible for someone to be unaware of the relationship between the spoken word and the printed symbol and that this is a fundamental weakness which has to be put right as a first priority.

By some, however, these sub-type names have come to be interpreted as though they stood for something permanent and immutable. This is to overlook the fact that Johnson and Myklebust were making a distinction *within* the area of verbal behaviour, and that there are subtle indications in their account of the educational treatment recommended that other factors are involved in the differences between the two groups besides modality; for instance it is members of the auditory dyslexic group, not the visual dyslexics, who may have to be taken back to recognizing the fundamental relationship between speech and the written language. In spite of this the assumption has sometimes been made that all that is necessary for deciding whether an individual is an auditory dyslexic or a visual dyslexic is to see whether he does worse on auditory or on visual tests. Then, if he is an auditory dyslexic (or 'visual learner') one uses 'visual' methods - that is, whole-word reading and 'look and say' - whereas if he is a visual dyslexic (or 'auditory learner') one uses 'auditory' methods - that is, associating letters with their sounds.

This practice, which represents a distortion of the views of Johnson and Myklebust, has been severely criticized by Liberman (1983). In this paper she begins by raising doubts about some of the tests which allegedly pick people out as being 'auditory' or 'visual' learners. One of the tests which has been used (or rather misused) for this purpose is the *Illinois Test of Psycholinguistic Abilities* (ITPA) (McCarthy and Kirk 1961). Liberman's discussion is not intended as a criticism of this test in general but is intended to show how easily an incautious user can draw wrong inferences. The following passage is worth quoting in full:

> The auditory reception sub-test is described as a test to 'assess the ability of a child to derive meaning from verbally presented material'. It takes the form of simple interrogatory sentences – 'Do dogs eat?', 'Do dials yawn?', 'Do wingless birds soar?' – which the child answers Yes or No. The difficulty of the task derives from the increasingly difficult level of the vocabulary used. In order to answer a question correctly the child must, of course, be familiar with its constituent words.
>
> (p. 4)

Another test, in contrast, is described as 'a measure of the child's ability to gain meaning from visual symbols'. The child is shown, for instance, a picture of a desk lamp and has to choose, from one of four pictures on the next page, 'the object or situation which is conceptually similar to the stimulus' – in this case a table lamp as opposed to a flashlight, light bulb, or lantern. Liberman continues:

> Now if we seek to determine the modality preference of a child from a pair of tests, we must surely demand that the two tests be similar in all respects except for the differences in modality. The auditory and visual subtests of receptive language of the ITPA obviously do not meet that criterion. To be sure, in one subtest, the items are presented auditorily and in the other visually, but there are many other differences which are not modality related. A question to be answered 'Yes' or 'No' is the test format in one, a multiple choice procedure in the other. Vocabulary level increases in difficulty in one and not in the other. Practical knowledge and abstract reasoning are central to one and not to the other.... In the face of all these differences that are not modally related, it stretches credulity to the snapping point to believe that such test pairs can determine the modality preference.
>
> (p. 5)

In her view the difficulties of poor readers are usually linguistic in origin, and this means that the search for 'auditory dyslexics' and 'visual dyslexics' is basically misguided.

The Aston Index (Newton and Thomson 1976) also makes use of the 'auditory–visual' distinction; and since some of its items are similar to those in the ITPA there are the same traps for the unwary: because a test is presented visually it does not follow that those who find it difficult can usefully be described as having 'visual' problems. Indeed it is sometimes supposed that the separate 'auditory' and 'visual' items of the Aston Index can be used to classify children into fixed 'types' with different teaching needs. Once again, however, the tests are not parallel, any more than are the ITPA ones. In addition we find on page 10 of *The Aston Portfolio* (Aubrey *et al.* 1980) that 'reversal problems' are listed among 'difficulties in visual skills'; and this, as we have already seen (Chapters 1 and 5), is an over-simplification.

At least some of the Aston group, however, appear to have modified this view. Thus Richards, another prominent member of the group, writes as follows:

> Reversal errors in reading and spelling are commonly supposed to be characteristic of visual difficulties but it has been shown that these may in fact represent a failure of the verbal mediation process, the dyslexic learner being unable to remember which label is associated with which symbol.
>
> (Richards 1985, pp. 37–8)

This seems to us a correct view of the situation. With the Aston Index, however, as with the work of Johnson and Myklebust, there is still a danger that some practising teachers will give more weight to the 'auditory'–'visual' distinction than the evidence warrants.

Another well-known attempt at sub-typing is that of Boder (1973). Dyslexics, on her view, can be classified as 'dysphonetic', 'dyseidetic' or 'mixed'. The first group are said to have a 'primary deficit in symbol–sound (grapheme–phoneme) integration, resulting in inability to develop phonetic word analysis–synthesis skills' (p. 667). The second group comprise 'children whose reading–spelling pattern reflects primary deficit in the ability to perceive letters and whole words as configurations or visual gestalts' (p. 667).

Boder's basic procedure can be summarized as follows. In the first place the child is presented with single words to read. If the word is recognized within one second an entry is made in a column marked 'flash'; if it is recognized within about 10 seconds the entry is made in a column marked 'untimed'. A preponderance of entries in the 'flash' column indicates that the child is reading by means of whole-word Gestalten, whereas a preponderance of words in the 'untimed' column indicates that he/she is reading by means of phonic analysis. Supporting evidence is looked for by means of a spelling test. Words in the child's sight vocabulary for reading ('flash' words) are presented orally and the child is asked to spell them, the results being compared with words which on the reading test were placed in the 'unknown' column; phonetic analysis skills are determined by the child's ability to spell 'unknown' words correctly.

However, when one examines Boder's examples of a 'dys-phonetic' type of pupil and a 'dyseidetic' type, one is surprised to find that the former is a 15-year-old boy with a Stanford-Binet IQ of 92, who has been in a special reading class for three years (what methods were they using?), while the other is a much younger boy, aged 8½ with an IQ of 145 – bursting, no doubt, to communicate somehow! It was surely unwise, to say the least, to use such cases as examples of 'two separate types' when all sorts of developmental factors could account for the reported differences, for instance, severity of handicap, intelligence, temperament, and stage in education.

It is interesting to note that confusions between 'b' and 'd' and other so-called 'reversal' errors were found by Boder in all three groups; she claims simply that they are more common in younger children (pp. 671–2). If such errors could, indeed, be described as visual, it is perhaps surprising that they were not more common in Boder's 'dyseidetic' group. If, however, as has been suggested above, the mistake is one at the level of language, this ceases to be a valid objection.

Evidence which appears to go against Boder's view has been published by van den Bos (1984). He classified a group of dyslexic children aged 9 and 10 according to her specification, and tested their memory for single letters in both visual and auditory conditions. No differences between the three groups were found. In addition it was noted by Miles (1983) that when he compared the performance of dyslexic subjects at recall of auditorily presented digits with their performance at recall of visually presented digits there was no evidence that those who were strong in the one condition tended to be weaker in the other. This finding, too, casts doubt on the value of Boder's classification.

A final attempt at sub-typing requires brief mention. Seymour (1986) writes as follows:

> For the purpose of discussing basic reading functions, it appeared to me to be minimally necessary to postulate central co-operating systems concerned with the representation of meaning and the representation of speech together with a system for the visual analysis and identification of print and writing. I will refer to the first two systems as a 'semantic processor' and a 'phonological processor'. The third system will be referred to as the 'visual (graphemic) processor'.
>
> (p. 13)

One of his main objectives was to study whether his dyslexic subjects consistently showed disorders in one or more of these systems. His method allowed for three choices:

> If developmental dyslexia is homogeneous all dyslexic cases will receive the same cognitive description.... If sub-types exist, there will be a small number of distinctively different descriptions, each shared by a number of individuals.... If the dyslexic population is heterogeneous each subject will receive a different cognitive description.
>
> (p. 9)

By a 'cognitive description' he means an account of what function or functions are impaired, given the processing systems postulated by his model.

His subjects were twenty-one dyslexics aged between 12 years 3 months and 25 years 3 months, all but two being in the average range of intelligence or above. Thirteen competent readers, aged between 10 years 9 months and 12 years 3 months, were used as controls. Among the dyslexics he found 'large differences in the distribution and extent of inefficiencies and in the choice of processing options' (p. 239), from which he concluded that there is no 'single adverse factor which produces a consistent set of impairments within the processing system' (pp. 239–40). Nor, in his view, can the data 'easily be fitted into a coherent scheme of sub-types' (p. 240).

Given his procedures, this outcome is not very surprising. Although he rightly criticizes some of the researchers in the field of acquired dyslexia for relying on single-case studies, his use of twenty-one subjects creates difficulties of its own. Since they varied considerably in both age and intelligence level, and some had reading ages at the top of the scale on the Schonell Word Recognition Test, it is likely that all kinds of developmental factors were influencing the results. He did, however, find evidence of phonological weakness in all his dyslexic subjects, in the sense of 'inaccuracy or reaction time delays in reading non-words' (p. 246). As for his 'visual processor dyslexia', this expression is perhaps something of a misnomer. He himself says that this is not equivalent to Boder's 'dyseidetic dyslexia' or to the 'visual dyslexia' of Stein and Fowler (see this book, Chapter 5); indeed four of his 'visual processor dyslexics' had fixed reference eyes, while two of his subjects with unfixed reference eye were not in fact classified as 'visual processor dyslexics'. The criterion which Seymour used for his classification was in fact a test of matching letter arrays, and it is by no means clear that visual processing is all that is involved in this task. As has been suggested in many places in this book, the display of seemingly 'visual' skills may in some cases be the consequence of ability to find the right name.

8

The question of sub-types II

This chapter will be concerned with the proposals for sub-typing which have arisen as a result of studies of acquired dyslexia.

When attempts were made, some fifteen years ago, to distinguish different syndromes of acquired dyslexia, the patients were classified into groups according to the types of reading or spelling errors that they made or the particular literacy skills that appeared to be lacking. Theories were then offered as to which particular function or 'route' had been put out of action. One of the earliest of such classifications was made by Marshall and Newcombe (1973), who picked out three types, namely 'visual dyslexia', 'deep dyslexia' and 'surface dyslexia'. Other types which have since been added, include 'direct dyslexia', 'attentional dyslexia' and 'phonological dyslexia' (for further details and an indication of what functions may be disturbed in each case see Marshall 1984 and A.W. Ellis 1984).

The question then arose as to whether anything analogous to these different sub-types was to be found in developmental dyslexia. If so, there would be a sound theoretical basis either for assimilating developmental dyslexia to a particular sub-type of acquired dyslexia or for saying that it, too, had a variety of sub-types.

For reasons which will be found in Marshall (1984), 'visual dyslexia', 'direct dyslexia' and 'attentional dyslexia' can be excluded from the present inquiry. This leaves deep dyslexia, surface dyslexia and phonological dyslexia.

Detailed discussions of deep dyslexia will be found in Coltheart *et al.* (1986). Some of the main characteristics of the deep dyslexic are (i) difficulty in reading non-words, that is, legitimate combinations of letters which do not form an existing word, for instance 'nate'; (ii) a tendency to make 'semantic' errors, for instance, in the absence of contextual cues, reading 'food' for 'dinner' or 'cousin' for 'uncle'; (iii) more difficulty in reading abstract (or non-imageable) words than concrete words, for example 'concept' as opposed to 'kettle'; and (iv) more difficulty in reading function words than content words, for instance 'be' as compared with 'bee'. To oversimplify somewhat, the argument is that the 'route' which allows for phonic analysis is damaged. This would make sense not only of the difficulty with non-words but would actually explain the very puzzling and challenging phenomenon of semantic errors, since if the 'route to meaning' is undamaged a word in the correct semantic category may be evoked even though its correctness cannot easily be checked by an examination of its component letters. Possible theoretical explanations of (iii) and (iv) are complex and need not concern us here, though it should be noted that relative difficulty with non-imageable words is not limited to poor readers (Baddeley *et al.* 1982).

Patients who are 'surface dyslexics' are a complete contrast, since they do not make semantic errors and are able to read non-words. Unlike deep dyslexics, however, they have a poor sight vocabulary. Moreover when they spell they tend simply to apply phoneme–grapheme correspondence rules, and a characteristic regularly found in their reading is the confusion of homophones, as when 'mare' is interpreted as the mayor of a town. The inference is that the route to whole-word representations is damaged: to quote Marshall (1984, p. 50), 'it is the phonologic representation (right or wrong) that determines the patient's semantic interpretation'.

The contrast between these two types of dyslexia is described by Marcel (1986, p. 227) as follows:

> When attempting to read single words, the nature of the errors made by deep dyslexic patients appears to be determined at least in part by the semantic and syntactic nature of the target word and semantic and syntactic processing of it. The nature of the errors made by surface dyslexic patients appears to be determined largely by spelling-to-sound characteristics of the target word.

'Phonological dyslexia' is a more recent addition to the list, and seems to be a less severe variant of 'deep dyslexia' which is found in a few cases. As in the latter, non-words are a problem, as are derivational errors, for instance misreading 'wise' as 'wisdom'. Also prefixes and suffixes are sometimes added, dropped, or substituted, for example 'thinking' for 'think', 'disposal' for 'dispose', or 'eradicate' for 'ineradicable'. However there is no particular preference shown for concrete or imageable words. Overall there are fewer errors over non-words than in the case of deep dyslexics and far fewer omissions (Sartori *et al.* 1984).

Whatever the parallels between developmental and acquired dyslexia there are some obvious dissimilarities. In particular the acquired dyslexic is one who has lost skills which previously he/she had gained in the normal way, whereas the developmental dyslexic never possessed them in the first place. It should be remembered, too, that the effects in adult life of a gunshot wound or a serious road accident are likely to be devastating, and they are also likely to be untidy in the sense of not being clearly circumscribed. In contrast, although it is important not to minimize the problems of a developmental dyslexic, developmental dyslexia is not a disaster on this massive scale. Moreover injuries to the brain of an adult are often permanently destructive of function, whereas there are good reasons for believing that developmental dyslexics can be successfully taught new skills (see Chapter 10). In addition, though there may be anomalies in the brain of a developmental dyslexic (see Chapter 3) these can be picked out only by very refined techniques. Finally, in their case years of development, even if somewhat abnormal compensatory development, and years of attempted teaching by one method or another must surely lead one to expect different performances at different ages. Indeed it is likely that some of the many differences between one developmental dyslexic and another are due to such developments, possibly on top of differences in the initial severity of the condition.

Nevertheless it is worth while reflecting further on possible similarities. We shall therefore comment on some of the research which has been carried out in this area. Since, however, this has so far involved only a limited number of developmental dyslexics, we have supplemented the more systematic evidence with generalizations and examples from our own experience.

There is no doubt (see Chapter 9) that many developmental dyslexics have phonological coding difficulties; to this extent they are similar to both phonological and deep dyslexics. It would not therefore be surprising if some of them were found to be poor at reading non-words, and this has in fact been shown to be the case (Jorm 1979). In contrast, the subjects studied by Baddeley *et al.* (1982) were fairly successful at this task, though they needed more time than the controls. The explanation of the discrepancy between these results seems to be that phonic skills can be *taught*, and indeed *are* taught at special units or at schools such as the one from which Baddeley *et al.* drew their dyslexic subjects. In general, if letter–sound correspondences are known and segmentation problems can be overcome it is by no means impossible for developmental dyslexics to read non-words, even though many of them may not be all that good at it.

There is no hard evidence in respect of semantic errors. It is a matter of familiar experience that, when contextual cues are present, many developmental dyslexics will try to use them, and, in so doing, may go wrong in a variety of ways, for instance by paraphrasing or producing synonyms. To take two examples from our own experience, a boy aged 11, along with various other errors in the same passage, read 'Sunday' for 'Saturday', while another, of the same age, read 'cuddle' for 'kiss'. In such cases, however, there is some degree of phonic similarity to the target word, and it would appear that there has been a limited amount of decoding even though this is not complete. Such decoding is precisely what is missing in the case of the semantic errors made by deep dyslexics. An apparent example of such an error came our way some years ago. This was a boy aged 10 who was attempting to read the word 'heroic' from the Schonell R1 Word Recognition Test (which involves presenting single words out of context). He said, 'I know that word – it means "brave"', doesn't it?', but failed to read it correctly. It is doubtful, however, if this was a genuine semantic error: a more likely explanation is that the boy had *partially* decoded the word and was therefore able to see the association with 'hero' but did not know, or could not call to mind, the related adjective, heroic – a word which not only is less frequent than the noun, 'hero', but differs from it in being stressed on the second syllable. In general, it would be correct to say, after many years' use of the Schonell R1 Word Recognition Test, that neither of us has met a single case of a semantic error similar to those made by deep dyslexics. If any subject had ever read, say, 'chemistry' in place of 'physics' (where there could not have been any partial decoding), the situation would have been different. As things are, most of the errors that we have met have been influenced by the context when the child is reading a continuous text.

With regard to function words and non-imageable words, it is regularly reported that developmental dyslexics are weak at getting 'little' words right. These words, of course, are often the ones for which the reader cannot easily get help from the context. Mistakes with such words, however, may simply be due to absence of phonic skills, and a dyslexic child is not likely to make a big effort to decode if he can get the sense of the sentence without doing so. Although the end product, therefore – a tendency to make errors over function words – is common to developmental and deep dyslexics, it is not clear that this similarity is of major significance.

Jorm (1979) maintained that developmental dyslexics were most like deep dyslexics because of the difficulties which both have with non-words. (Phonological dyslexia had not been mentioned at that time.) Others, however, have argued that a better comparison can be made with surface dyslexia (Baddeley *et al*. 1982; Temple and Marshall 1983; Coltheart *et al*. 1983; Temple 1985; Baddeley *et al*. 1988). The argument, in brief, is that surface dyslexics are known to be able to make use of letter–sound correspondences (the postulated 'route' being undamaged) and that, unlike deep dyslexics, they are therefore able to read non-words. Similarly, it would be said, developmental dyslexics make fewer mistakes with regular words than with irregular ones, and, unlike deep dyslexics, are at least *capable* of reading non-words even though some of them find it difficult to do so.

In the case of phonological dyslexia, it might seem at first glance that the similarities with developmental dyslexia are obvious. Let us take as an example the reading errors made by the phonological dyslexic, A.M., as reported by Patterson (1982). A.M., who had suffered a thrombosis, was reported as having difficulty in letter naming, and in addition made numerous small errors in reading single words from the Schonell R1 Word Recognition test. These included 'applause' for 'applaud', 'situate' for 'situated', 'fascinating' for 'fascinate', and 'judiciary' for 'judicature'. Certainly, on the face of it, these are just the sort of errors that a developmental dyslexic might make, many of them being so-called 'derivational' errors, for instance reading a noun for the corresponding verb, as in the case of 'applause', or supplying an incorrect verb form, as in 'fascinating'. Even here, however, it is important not to overlook the differences.

Experience suggests that many developmental dyslexics are not explicitly aware of grammatical distinctions which other children easily pick up – between a noun and a verb, for instance, or between a participle and a past tense. Lacking this knowledge they may fail to notice differences in bound morphemes (–ed, –ing, etc.) and hence make errors which seem similar to those made by A.M. One must suppose that in his case, however, he lacked the phonic skills needed for making the necessary small adjustments. It is even possible that the words which he produced may have been more familiar in his past reading than the words which were actually in front of him, and that this may have influenced his responses. From Patterson's account he had been a very literate man before his accident, and one should therefore be cautious in drawing parallels between his errors and those made by people who could achieve comparable standards of literacy, if at all, only after a considerable struggle.

Overall, then, it may be doubted if these alleged similarities are of major significance for our understanding of developmental dyslexia. In this connection Marshall (1984) writes as follows: 'Intuitively I feel that it is really quite unlikely that the acquired and developmental dyslexias will be interpretable over a single static functional architecture' (i.e. a diagram of functions which does not change over time). He continues: 'There should, I suspect, be some qualitative changes in functional architecture that arise both in the normal growth of reading skill and in consequence of developmental impairments' (p. 55). This is important advice and should warn us against looking for too close parallels. Yet it seems that Temple (1985) made precisely this mistake in her account of a 12-year-old boy (S.L.). Having noted that he produced errors about half the time which showed some elementary knowledge of grapheme–phoneme correspondence, she concluded that he was 'a developmental surface dyslexic with impairment of the parser and the translator' (Temple 1985, p. 282). One feels that it might have been more profitable to say simply that there were certain skills which S.L. had not yet learned. It is also important to bear in mind the point made by Bryant and Impey (1987), viz. that if the intention is to explain the specific difficulties of developmental dyslexics, it makes no sense to invoke error patterns which also occur in normal readers.

There is, indeed, good evidence, as will be seen in Chapter 9, that developmental dyslexics show weakness at associating letters with the corresponding sounds, which means that, to this extent at least, they are unlike surface dyslexics. Moreover, in view of this weakness it is not surprising that they should at least be *slow* at reading non-words (Baddeley *et al.* 1982). On this basis one could argue either that they are like deep dyslexics because they find the reading of non-words difficult, or that they are unlike them because some of them find it possible. To say that they are either 'like' or 'unlike' without qualification is therefore an oversimplification.

The point of most importance is that one should not overlook the part played by developmental factors as children learn to read; this of itself should alert us to the fact that any comparison must have its limitations. In particular, if research is carried out at schools which offer special provision for dyslexics, it is virtually certain that such dyslexics will be being taught letter-sound correspondences in a systematic way. Much may therefore depend on how long the teaching has been going on and what stage they have reached. Those who have not been exposed to such teaching or have made little progress may well find the reading of non-words difficult, whereas those with the appropriate experience may be reasonably successful.

Similarly, in investigations of spelling, one may well meet the occasional dyslexic who spells phonetically; that is to say, he uses the limited number of spelling patterns that he knows in order to reproduce the sounds of the words that he needs. However, teachers of dyslexics know only too well that it is very easy to turn one who is originally phonologically very weak into a speller of this kind by unremitting phonic instruction; it is an attainable target for both teacher and pupil, and at least it enables the pupil to communicate. It is therefore quite conceivable that a child who is a mild case of developmental dyslexia might settle for phonetic spelling without systematic teaching. It is certainly reported that the Danish dyslexic, Edith Norrie, taught herself to read and spell that way and was able to invent a specially arranged 'phonological' system to help others (for further reference to the Edith Norrie Letter Case see Chapter 10). There is much to motivate someone with a good oral vocabulary to proceed phonetically in order to communicate rather than to attempt to become a fully accurate speller. One must constantly remember that the dyslexic has had to devise compensatory strategies of *some* kind, and these compensatory strategies could mistakenly be interpreted as permanent type characteristics.

It is not in dispute that the search for parallels between developmental and acquired dyslexia has generated some interesting research and that certain similarities with all three types (deep, surface and phonological) have emerged. The final word, however, must be one of caution. The question, 'What route is damaged?', is a perfectly proper one if such damage is likely to have permanent effects. In the case of developmental dyslexics, however, the growth factor needs to be taken into account: with suitable teaching there is a great deal that they can learn. To divide them into fixed and by implication permanent types is to overlook the fact that they learn new skills over time.

9
Phonological deficits

At the end of Chapter 1 we raised some doubts about the correctness of the visually orientated interpretations of dyslexia put forward by Hinshelwood and Orton. For the last two decades the difficulties in this approach have been increasingly emphasized (see in particular Vellutino 1979 and Calfs 1989). The present chapter gives some of the evidence that an approach via phonology is likely to be more profitable. By 'phonology' is meant the science of speech sounds in so far as they convey meaning, while 'phonological processing' refers to operations by which stimuli are interpreted in terms of the speech sounds involved. Dyslexia, on this showing, is not a disorder of vision or of spatial orientation but a subtle kind of disorder in the area of language.

An important lead in shifting to more emphasis on a linguistic approach was given by Professor Isabelle Liberman and her colleagues at the University of Connecticut and the Haskins Laboratories. One of their early papers is worth describing in detail (Liberman *et al.* 1971). At the start of this paper the authors suggest the following questions for investigation: (i) whether 'reversals' are characteristic of beginning readers in general; (ii) what proportion of the errors can be classified as 'reversals'; (iii) what the relation is between 'kinetic' reversals (reversals of letter order) and 'static' reversals (orientational reversals), and, finally, (iv) whether reversals in reading are simply a problem in visual perception, as had been assumed, or whether there was a need to consider also the linguistic function of the letter shapes. The subjects in this investigation were 59 second-grade children of whom 18 (the lowest third in scores on a 60-word reading test) were selected for further study. They were aged between 7 years 3 months and 9 years 3 months; 15 were boys and 3 were girls, and all were within the IQ range 85–126 on the Wechsler Intelligence Scale for Children. After this initial selection they were given a further reading test and a task involving the matching of single letters to the correct member of a group of five letters, viz. 'b', 'd', 'p', 'g' and 'e'. All these letters, except the last, were assumed to be 'reversible'. The errors in both tasks were divided into four categories, viz. reversal of sequence, reversal of orientation, other consonant errors, and vowel errors. When the figures for all the children given the initial reading test were analysed it was found that nearly all the mistakes in the first two categories occurred among the 18 poor readers. What was particularly striking, however, was that these so-called 'reversal' errors accounted for only a small proportion of the misread letters. The figures were as follows:

Reversal of sequence	10%
Reversal of orientation	15%
Other consonant errors	32%
Vowel errors	43%

The analysis also showed that the number of reversals varied considerably from one child to another, that there was no correlation between 'static' and 'kinetic' reversals, and that confusions between reversible letters rarely occurred when these were presented singly, that is, out of context. They conclude with the suggestion that 'further exploration of the linguistic determination of children's errors is likely to be profitable' (Liberman *et al.* 1971, p. 141).

This evidence shows at the very least that mistakes which could be classified as 'reversals' are relatively infrequent; and it is possible therefore that their importance has been over emphasized. Evidence from other sources also points to a similar conclusion (see Hulme 1981, Chapter 1).

Moreover, once it has been shown that the great majority of letter errors committed by retarded readers cannot be explained simply as visual errors, the door is then opened to other possible explanations of errors in 'reversible' letters too. For instance, confusion between 'b' and 'p' might be due more to auditory similarity than to visual similarity, since they are the voiced and unvoiced forms of the same plosive; or, again, it is possible that the differences between 'd' and 'b' may be obscured by unclear speech, since although these two letters are not very close auditorily they are close in their places of articulation. There is also the possibility of confusion in letter production in writing, a fact of which teachers are perhaps more likely to be conscious than neurologists: thus, since 'd' is the 'odd one out' among letters with uprights, in that the upright should be made last rather than first as one moves from left to right on the page, a child not noticing this and starting 'd' in the same place as he starts 'b' may quite easily produce a 'b' instead. Moreover, if a letter which comes out 'wrong' is not immediately corrected the confusion may become a habit, with the result that there is a nagging uncertainty whenever the letters have to be read or written. This could be similar to the 'cross-association' un-certainty discussed by Quinault (1972) who points out that many people hesitate, for instance, between 'port' and 'starboard' or between 'stalagmites' and 'stalactites'; provided both members of a pair are known it is very easy to confuse them and to have to ask oneself 'Which is which?'

Similarly there may be alternative explanations of 'reversals of sequence'. For example, if a child has not noticed that the 'ai' combination is pronounced as a long 'a' sound whereas the 'ia' combination is pronounced as two distinct vowels, as in 'dial', it is not surprising if he sometimes writes 'brian' in place of 'brain'. Nothing is gained by calling this a 'reversal' error, and to do so may even divert attention from the real source of his difficulty.

In a further study (Liberman *et al.* 1974), an attempt was made to examine the difficulties involved in segmenting speech into its constituent phonemes. Now in spoken language, although there are some acoustic criteria in the form of energy peaks which indicate where syllables divide, there are no such criteria to indicate where phonemes divide. In the words of the authors, 'To recover the phonemes from the sound into which they are so complexly encoded requires a decoder which segments the continuous acoustic signal according to linguistic rules' (ibid., p. 204). To test children's ability in this respect they compared 46 pre-school children (mean age 59 months), 49 children at kindergarten (mean age 70 months), and 40 children at first-grade level (mean age 83 months) in their ability to learn syllabic and phonemic segmentation. The task was to tap out the number of syllables or phonemes (after the experimenter had given examples of what was required) in a random arrangement of words containing three, two, or one syllables or three, two, or one phonemes. The criterion of success was the ability to tap out six consecutive items without any intervening demonstration by the experimenter. In all the groups segmentation into syllables turned out to be easier than segmentation into phonemes: thus 46 per cent of the pre-school children reached criterion for segmentation by syllables, but none could segment by phonemes; the figures for the kindergarten children were 48 per cent and 17 per cent, and for the first-grade children 90 per cent and 70 per cent.

The relation of this segmentation skill to reading progress has been highlighted by a much larger research project conducted by Bryant and Bradley of Oxford University (see Bradley and Bryant 1978, 1983; Bryant and Bradley 1985). Their project involved 368 children aged either 4 or 5 years, none of whom had yet shown any sign of reading. These children were tested on their ability to pick the 'odd one out' from three or four spoken words, all but the target word having a sound in common. Trials were made with the end sound (bun *hut* gun sun), the middle sound (*hug* pig dig wig), and the beginning sound (bud bun bus *rug*). Three or four years later the results of these tests were found to correlate highly with the children's scores on a reading test (single-word recognition) and on a spelling test, even when, by a suitable statistical technique, differences in intelligence were allowed for. Next the authors conducted a training study involving 65 of these children who at the age of 6 years had made no progress in reading and had the lowest segmentation scores. The children in one group were presented with pictures and given practice at picking out the sounds which the picture-names had in common; in a second group the procedure was the same but in addition the children were trained to use plastic letters corresponding to the sounds; in a third group (to control for possible Hawthorne effects) the children were given an equal amount of attention but were trained to classify by meaning (for instance, 'hen' and 'bat' as animals, 'hen' and 'pig' as farm animals, etc.), while a fourth group received no training at all. The first two groups made the most progress (the second group being slightly ahead of the first group), and there were no significant differences between the third and fourth groups. Although the differences between the groups were not large, they were invariably in the predicted direction; and the actual amount of training (40 short sessions over a 2-year period) is less than that available to many remedial teachers. There is thus good evidence of a relationship between ability to categorize sounds and ability to read.

There is an interesting connection between this research and the model proposed by Frith (1985). Frith divides the development of reading into three stages, which she terms 'logographic', 'alphabetic' and 'orthographic'. In the first stage the child makes a rough and ready response to written words on a pattern recognition basis. Since this method soon turns out to be inadequate the child next tries to develop alphabetic skills. These involve the implicit knowledge that individual phonemes can be represented by single letters (or sometimes by digraphs); and it then becomes possible for the child to analyse the word into its components, to write down the letters of phonetically regular words, and to read nonsense words. Finally, in the orthographic stage, the child learns to identify words at sight, though at this stage she may be able to use her alphabetic skills as a fall-back.

Now it seems likely that the typical dyslexic child is held up at the alphabetic stage: in some cases he may not even be aware that written letters correspond to sounds, and even when he has learned or been taught this the correct 'pairing' is by no means easy for him and is likely to require many repetitions. (We shall be noting in Chapter 10 how in their teaching system Gillingham and Stillman insist on the thorough learning of 'linkages'.) Failure to pass through the alphabetic stage may result in inappropriate strategies at a later age, for instance trying to rely on a none too efficient memory in order to recall individual letters, with no understanding of what function these letters are performing or why they occur in a particular order. As was suggested above, it is possible that what Orton called 'kinetic reversals' can more usefully be interpreted in this way. Failure to develop and use alphabetic skills can result in children perceiving the task of learning to read as one of committing to memory visual units, using whatever visual features seem most serviceable for this purpose (Stuart and Coltheart 1988). Yet if unfamiliar words are to be read, let alone spelled, such memorizing will be insufficient, and mastery of the alphabetic code will be a necessity.

Similarly, when Rack (1985) compared twelve 14-year-old dyslexics with younger children matched for reading age on a set of rhyming tasks ('farm'/'calm', 'farm'/'warm', 'head'/'said', etc.) there were no differences in error rate, but the dyslexics were slower and tended to make greater use of the orthographic characteristics of the word. This result supplies further confirmation that dyslexics are at a disadvantage as compared with other children when dealing with the relationship between speech sounds and written or printed letters and in particular may find it more difficult to blend speech sounds when faced with an unfamiliar word in reading.

Another area of difficulty for dyslexics seems to be that of producing the right name. Even when the stimulus is something completely familiar such as a strip of colour or the picture of a familiar object the time needed to 'find' the appropriate word appears to be longer (Spring and Capps 1974; Done and Miles 1988). In a particularly interesting study Denckla and Rudel (1976) made a comparison between 10 children with reading difficulty and 10 children who showed learning difficulties of other kinds, for instance attention deficits, problems with mathematics, or problems with handwriting, even though they had no marked difficulty with reading. These children, along with 90 others of the same age range (8 to 10 years), were given a picture naming test, which had originally been devised by Oldfield and Wingfield (1965) for dysphasic adults and had then been adapted by themselves for use with children. What particularly impressed the authors was not the comparative numbers of errors but the circumlocutions and phonetically distorted yet recognizable replies which were given by the dyslexics, as against the completely incorrect identifications characteristic of the other learning difficulties group. It was also found that on the Peabody Picture Vocabulary Test the poor readers came out with scores which were above the average for that of the 90 controls. This result is not in fact surprising if one remembers that in this test the subjects themselves do not have to produce words; their task is to point to the correct picture, from a choice of four, when someone else supplies the name. Difficulties in the actual finding of the right word are therefore not an obstacle to obtaining a high score.

It was noted in the last chapter how the reading of nonsense words often presented difficulty to developmental dyslexics. This task requires both the phonological encoding of visual marks and the blending of the resultant sounds, and it has to be carried out in a context where there is no possibility of guessing the word on the basis of incomplete information, as there is in the case of real words. An interesting variant is to present non-words auditorily. It should be noted in this connection that non-words are not simply 'environmental sounds', since if they are to be remembered they need to be phonologically represented no less than do real words or visually presented non-words. In an experiment carried out by Done and Miles (1978), ten dyslexic subjects, aged 14, were compared with a 'matched pair' control in a paired-associate learning task. One set of stimuli comprised visually presented nonsense shapes; the other set comprised nonsense words based on three-letter trigrams (consonant-vowel-consonant). Five such pairs of stimuli were used, and, after an introductory run in which the subjects were told the 'names' of the shapes, they had to say them aloud as each shape was presented, the correct 'name' being given immediately afterwards. A record was kept of the number of trials needed by the subject in order to produce two consecutive error-free runs. The figures for the ten matched pairs were as follows:

Pair number	1	2	3	4	5	6	7	8	9	10
Control subjects	11	17	12	6	10	13	11	13	16	11
Dyslexic subjects	31	8	29	30	17	41	46	24	18	20

With one exception, therefore, the dyslexics needed more trials than the controls before the associations were formed. This procedure is in some ways a replication of the situation which occurs when a child first learns to talk, since what were initially mere 'sounds' become linked with particular features in the environment. As will be seen later, weakness at building up phonological representations and weakness at paired-associate learning seem to be part and parcel of the same phenomenon.

In an interesting set of experiments Katz (1986) presented his subjects with a series of pictures, of graded difficulty, for which they had to produce the correct name. He found a significant correlation between reading level and error rate; and he was able to show that this was not due to lack of familiarity with the objects or their names, since the same result was obtained when he used only those words which the children immediately recognized when he himself produced the name. In a second experiment, after it had been checked that the subjects could distinguish rhyming and non-rhyming words presented orally, they were required to press one or other of two keys according to whether or not the objects shown in two pictures had names which rhymed; and again the poor readers were inferior. The same subjects were also asked to respond by pressing one of two keys according to whether or not the names of two objects in a picture were both 'short' (i.e. monosyllabic); and it was found that the poor readers were inferior on this task even when they were able to give the name of the object afterwards. From these experiments it seemed to Katz that not only did the poor readers show difficulty in representing phonological information fully, but also in using accurately represented information to make linguistic judgements. Although Katz's 'poor readers' were in fact only poor readers in comparison to their classmates, since they were at or not much below grade level, it is noteworthy that even with this relatively mild degree of retardation their performance was significantly different from that of the better readers.

Stirling and Miles (1988) have also produced evidence which seems to confirm that dyslexics have difficulties with oral language. Their subjects were 21 dyslexic boys aged between the ages of 12 and 16 years and 19 age-matched controls. In their first experiment the subjects were asked to produce the name of the particular part of a picture, for instance the *buckle* of a shoe or the *hand* of a watch. In untimed conditions the dyslexics produced as many correct answers as did the controls, but some of the words were distorted, for example one of them said 'bucker' in place of 'buckle' and two of them said 'handle' in place of 'hand'. In a second experiment the subjects were presented orally with words which they were required to define. Some of these words had two meanings, being either homographs (such as 'vice'/'vice') or homophones (such as 'peer'/'pier'), the original purpose of the experiment being to check whether the dyslexics could 'shift' from one meaning of a homonym or homophone to the other. In this respect they were in fact no different from the controls; but they showed some curious distortions and misapprehensions, including grammatical errors and incorrect verb forms. Thus in reply to 'peer' ('pier') one boy said 'I appear to look for something', while another said 'A pier is what people walk along and fishing off'; in response to 'vice' one boy said 'Someone to help you, give you advice', while another said 'A vice is like something you give'; 'crocus' was defined as 'a plant, or a game' (croquet!), and in response to 'chip' one boy said, 'A chip is – er – you can give a chip to a waiter or something like that . . . you give him a chip, you sort of chip'.

Another study (Snowling *et al.* 1986) suggests that dyslexics are weak not only at the explicit analysis of the acoustic information needed for reading and spelling but even at carrying out analysis at the level necessary for accurate repetition of words and non-words. Their subjects were 19 disabled readers, 19 normal readers of similar chronological age and intelligence, and 19 younger children of similar reading age and intelligence. Words were presented orally, and the subject's task was to repeat them. On high-frequency words there were no differences between the groups; on low-frequency words the performance of the disabled readers was worse than that of the age-matched controls but not worse than that of the reading-age-matched controls, while on the non-words it was worse than that of both other groups. In a further experiment the same children listened to a mixture of words and non-words and had to say in each case whether it was a real word or not. Here, too, the disabled readers were inferior to the age-matched controls, but in this case they performed at much the same level as did the reading-age controls. One must assume that over the years the dyslexics had been exposed sufficiently often to the high-frequency words for these words to have become firmly established and thus readily available. With low-frequency words, however, and even more with nonsense words the time needed for 'retrieval' was longer, and fewer words could therefore be reproduced per unit time. What appears to be involved here, as the authors point out, is a link between difficulties at the phonological level and problems with short-term memory. It is to this issue that we must now turn.

There is, of course, a very extensive literature on memory in general, and we shall limit ourselves to a discussion of theories and research that are relevant to the issue of dyslexia.

It is not easy to summarize without oversimplification. In brief, however, it can be said that since the late 1950s it has been widely agreed that a distinction can usefully be drawn between 'long-term memory' and 'short-term memory'. In this context a 'short-term' memory task is one where the delay between the presentation of the stimulus is a matter of seconds rather than any longer time interval. It does not, of course, follow that there are just two 'memory systems', one for long-term tasks and one for short-term tasks; the matter is clearly more complicated than this. It was originally found useful, however – though even this is an oversimplification (see below) – to hypothesize that in long-term memory words are coded semantically – that is, according to meaning – whereas in short-term memory the coding is phonological – that is, in terms of speech sounds. (Those wishing for further details may like to consult Baddeley 1976.)

Before we proceed further, a brief mention should be made of so-called 'iconic' memory. In a classic experiment it was shown by Sperling (1960) that when subjects are presented with a visual display they are able to respond to the properties of the stimulus for a brief period of time – perhaps 150 ms – after the display has been turned off. This led researchers to postulate a very simple system, the 'iconic' store, in which visual material was retained in its original form before further processing took place. It is convenient, as far as the present discussion is concerned, to deal with the iconic store at the outset, since its relevance to dyslexia in fact appears to be minimal. Under the influence of Sperling's original experiment several researchers surmised that the time during which the visual record was available in the iconic store might be different in the case of dyslexics – either because it lasted an extra long time with the result that the superimposition of after-images caused confusion, or because it did not last long enough and there was thus insufficient time to transfer the material into a more permanent store. Details of the techniques for measuring 'iconic storage' time need not concern us. Research in so far as it is relevant to dyslexia has been comprehensively reviewed by Vellutino (1979), who found that many of the results were negative and that none were fully convincing. There is thus little reason to believe that dyslexics differ from controls in 'iconic storage' time. This conclusion provides further support for the view that if one is looking for characteristics which distinguish dyslexics from non-dyslexics these are not likely to be found if one considers only the visual properties of the stimulus. The issue of iconic storage can therefore be excluded from further consideration.

Much recent research has been concerned in particular with the area of short-term memory, or 'working memory', as it is now often called. A very readable account of the main issues will be found in Baddeley (1986). In this book he describes working memory as 'a system for the temporary holding and manipulation of information during the performance of a range of cognitive tasks such as comprehension, learning, and reasoning' (p. 34). Later he describes how he and his colleague, Graham Hitch, abandoned the view of working memory as a single unitary store. We substituted the idea of a number of subsystems controlled by a limited capacity executive system.... We ... chose to operate initially with a tripartite system, comprising a supervisory controlling system, the *Central Executive*, aided by two slave systems, one of which was specialized for processing language material, the *Articulatory Loop*, and the other concerned with visuo–spatial memory, the *Visuo-Spatial Scratch Pad or Sketch Pad.*

(pp. 70–1)

We shall not be concerned in what follows with the 'visuo-spatial scratch pad', partly because dyslexics do not appear to have any marked difficulty in visuo-spatial tasks and partly because research in this area is not yet very far advanced. The system which is of most relevance for present purposes is that of the articulatory loop.

Now the fact that it is phonological features which are coded in short-term memory had been neatly demonstrated some years previously by Conrad (1964). Conrad studied the errors made by his subjects (who were normal readers) when they attempted to recall visually presented sequences of consonants. He found that when mistakes were made the letter chosen was often one that *sounded like* the correct one; thus 'B' was recorded as 'C', 'P', 'T', or 'V' far more often than it was recorded as 'F', 'M', 'N', 'S', or 'X'. This 'phonemic similarity effect' suggests that even when a stimulus is presented visually its phonological representation is what is memorized.

Another important short-term memory phenomenon is that of the 'word length effect' (Baddeley *et al.* 1975). In brief, if one is asked to remember a list of short words, such as 'sum', 'wit', 'hate', and so on, one can reproduce more of them than if the list contains longer words such as 'opportunity', 'university', 'aluminium', and so on. It is, of course, important that those who carry out research into the properties of words should be sure that they have controlled for all properties which might be affecting the result; for example, there is an overlap between long words, less frequent words, and words acquired later in life, and one cannot therefore claim that, say, frequency is the decisive factor without taking steps to rule out the influence of other factors. In this particular case there is reason to believe that the decisive factor is not the number of letters in the word or even the number of syllables but the time needed to say the word (Baddeley 1986, p. 80). This can be shown if one compares the results for two-syllable words some of which take longer to say than others, for instance 'harpoon' or 'Friday' as compared with 'bishop' or 'wicket'. The time over which items can be held in the articulatory loop has been reckoned to be about 1.7 seconds. An interesting discovery in this connection has been reported by Ellis and Hennelly (1980), viz. that native Welsh speakers could recall a larger number of digits when these were presented auditorily in English than when they were presented auditorily in Welsh, the reason, it seems, being that Welsh digit names take longer to pronounce.

Now there is good evidence that the 'phonemic similarity effect' is much less marked in dyslexics than in normal readers. Thus, in one experiment (Olson *et al.* 1984) 141 disabled readers, aged betwen 7 and 17, each with a matched control, were required to read a series of familiar words, some of which rhymed (for instance 'know', 'go') and some of which did not (for instance 'year', 'best'). They were then given a fresh list, containing some words from the original list and some new ones. They were asked to read the words in the second list silently and respond 'yes' or 'no' as quickly as possible according to whether the word was or was not in the first list. One of the interesting discoveries that came to light from an analysis of the errors made was a positive correlation among the disabled readers between age level and tendency to be influenced by rhyme; no such correlation was found among the controls. It seems reasonable to conclude in general that younger dyslexics are less influenced by the phonological features of the stimulus than are older dyslexics (compare also the experiments by Rack, 1985, mentioned above).

Finally, the following experiments by Torgesen and Houck (1980) point in the same direction. They selected three groups of 10-year-olds, with eight children in each, in the following way: one group (the 'N' group) comprised normal achievers; one comprised learning-disabled children with normal digit-span scores (the 'LD-N' group), and one comprised learning-disabled children with low digit-span scores (the 'LD-S' group). A variety of other tasks were given, besides recall of digits; and as a result the authors were able to rule out lack of attention, inadequate strategies, rate of presentation, and so on, as explanations of the weakness of the children in the LD-S group at this task. One of their most significant findings, however, was that when they presented their subjects visually with digits and then with pictures of animals and measured the response latencies in supplying the names there was a high correlation between the two sets of response latencies; and they conclude (p. 156) that 'the findings ... provide qualified support for the hypothesis that differences in rate of access to name codes for digits may underlie part of the difference in recall between LD-S children and those in the other two groups'. Cumulatively these and other experiments give strong support for the view that dyslexics show distinctive weakness at the phonological level.

It is perhaps also suggestive that there appear to be fewer literacy problems in Japan if children are taught *kanjis*, which are pictorial representations, than if they are taught the *kana*, which are phonetic symbols representing syllables. Clearly the reading of *kana* involves both phonological representation and the ability to synthesize words from their components; and if the 'phonological deficit' account of dyslexia is correct future research may well show that some Japanese children experience more difficulty with such reading than with the reading of *kanjis*. (For a discussion of this issue and an account of existing evidence see Thomson 1984, p. 116–18.)

At this point it may be useful to carry out a kind of stock-taking with regard to what it is that dyslexics find difficult. In this connection we shall be referring not only to the evidence cited in the present chapter but to that given in Chapter 6. We know that their memory span for both auditorily and visually presented digits is weak, that they are weak at phonemic segmentation, that they need many exposures before they can be successful at paired-associate learning, that they show uncertainty over 'left' and 'right', that they are slow at word finding, that they distort words in speech and cannot easily put the syllables in the correct order, that they do not easily learn number facts, and that some of them have difficulties with musical notation. How disparate, then, are these phenomena, and how far can they be accounted for in terms of a single theory?

Three of the key concepts appear to be weakness at the phonological level, weakness at paired-associate learning, and limited short-term memory. These are not rival 'theories of dyslexia', however; they should rather be seen as alternative formulations for describing what are largely the same facts.

Weakness at the phonological level covers much the same findings as weakness at paired-associate learning: one can accommodate both by saying that dyslexics have difficulty in associating events in the environment – and no doubt abstract ideas also – with their phonological representations. The important point here, of course, is not that this is impossible but that more pairings are needed before it is achieved; and it is perhaps for this reason more than for any other that comparisons between developmental dyslexia and acquired dyslexia are of limited value, since exposing acquired dyslexics to an increased number of paired associates is unlikely to be of much help to them. This may not, of course, be an *efficient* way of helping developmental dyslexics to learn things but it is at least a possible one if those concerned are prepared to put in sufficient time and effort. Weakness at paired-associate learning also makes sense of the difficulties experienced by dyslexics in learning number facts. Thus relatively few of them, unless they receive a highly traditional education in which recitation of tables is a daily task over many years, are likely, without calculation, to know, for instance, that 8 × 7 = 56; and if a basic knowledge of number facts is lacking there can be no opportunity for further 'paired-associate learning' (whether in class or to themselves privately) which would result in the acquisition of a wider range of number facts. In view of this weakness it would seem to be wise policy, when teaching either mathematics or music to dyslexics, to start with activity – *doing* subtraction, multiplication, and so on or *making* music – and only later try to teach them the relevant notation.

Difficulty in paired association may also make sense of the dyslexic's difficulty with the 'space' words, 'left', 'right', 'east' and 'west', and with the 'time' words, 'before' and 'after'. It may be surmised that these words are difficult because they do not *consistently* refer to any one feature in the environment; thus a hill that is 'on the left' when one is in a particular place may be 'on the right' if one is in another place. It is an obvious fact that even non-dyslexics sometimes make mistakes on such matters, but those who are any way weak at phonological representation can be expected to find this particular kind of phonological representation extra difficult.

It remains to consider in more detail the link between phonological weakness and poor short-term memory. The following description would seem to make good sense of the existing evidence. It is known that dyslexics need more time than non-dyslexics when the task is to supply the name of a colour or of an object; and it is therefore a reasonable surmise, particularly in view of the experiments of Torgesen and Houck (1980) (see above), that they will also need more time than non-dyslexics to convert an auditorily presented digit into its phonological representation. Since, however, the articulatory loop is one of limited capacity and fewer digits are being coded by dyslexics per unit time, it follows that their span for auditorily presented digits will necessarily be less. Moreover there is no reason why the position should be any different in the case of visually presented digits, since here, too, phonological representation would be needed.

The relationship between phonological deficiency and poor short-term memory has been neatly expressed by Vellutino (1987, p. 20); on his view what the deficiency involves is 'inability to represent and access the sound of a word in order to help remember the word'. If we think of each individual as possessing an internal 'lexicon' (or dictionary), we can then say that, as a person's language experience increases, more 'lexical entries' are acquired and become available for use. Developmental dyslexia could in that case be thought of as a family of weaknesses affecting the lexicon. These weaknesses would have various consequences. In the first place, more 'exposures' would be needed before appropriate 'lexical entries' could be built up; secondly, even when built up these entries would be less secure and more subject to distortion, while thirdly, even when they are secure and not distorted, they would still take longer to 'retrieve'. This kind of picture will undoubtedly need modification as research progresses, but one can fairly claim that it accommodates quite a large number of the facts which are already known. Finally, it needs to be emphasized that these weaknesses can be present not only when the visual system is intact but, more interestingly, when conceptual understanding and creativity are extremely high.

10

Teaching methods and programmes

Hinshelwood (1917) wrote as follows:

> My long experience of congenital word-blindness has enabled me to give with confidence a much more hopeful prognosis... viz. that in nearly all cases... the children so affected with proper treatment and great perseverance can be taught to read.... Such cases are the exact analogues of the conditions we have met with in acquired word-blindness due to disease. If in these latter cases, where the visual word centre has been destroyed, we have been able to re-educate such patients and enable them to regain the power of reading, then we have every reason to anticipate with confidence that in congenital cases, where the same centre is involved, a similar result will be accomplished by similar methods.
>
> (pp. 90-1)

Hinshelwood believed that what was involved was 'defect of the visual memory' (p. 105). Consequently:

> Education of the corresponding centre in the opposite side of the brain has to be accomplished just as in cases of acquired word-blindness.... We saw that all the cerebral centres concerned in language are ultimately connected with one another, and that experience has taught that the impressions made on one cerebral centre are deepened and strengthened by being associated with the impressions made on the other centres. Hence in the cases where we have a defective visual centre but the other cerebral centres intact, that method of instruction will in my opinion be the best in which a simultaneous appeal is made to other centres beside the visual. This condition is fulfilled by the old-fashioned

method of learning to read in which a simultaneous appeal is made
to visual centre, auditory centre and the centre for the memory of
speech movements.

(p. 105)

He also recommends the use of block letters, as by the constant
handling of these, so he found, 'the visual impressions were
strengthened by the simultaneous associations with the tactile
ones' (p. 106). It is interesting to note that, some 60 years later,
Hulme (1981) carried out systematic experiments on the effect of
tracing letters as an aid to remembering them and confirmed its
effectiveness. It is, of course, quite possible to carry out such
procedures without any theoretical commitment to belief in any
specific role for 'cerebral centres'; and Hinshelwood was not the
first person, nor will he be the last, to try to justify what is in fact
an effective method of teaching on the basis of some questionable
physiology.

One further point with regard to his views on teaching should
perhaps be noted. His emphasis on vision led him to suppose that
the 'auditory memory' was unimpaired. Indeed, he makes clear
that he is talking throughout about cases where the defect is
confined to the 'visual memory centre only' (p. 108). In later
teaching systems it is assumed, not that one 'centre' is weak and
all others are strong, but that inputs through the different
sensory channels mutually support each other. Hinshelwood's
proposals, therefore, though in some ways an anticipation of
what we now call 'multisensory teaching', were in this important
respect different from it. If he had known that many of his pupils
were weak at the recall of auditorily presented digits (as it is
virtually certain they would have been), he might well have been
led to revise his theory.

Orton's views on teaching were in some ways similar to those
of Hinshelwood. The work of developing remedial techniques
consistent with his working hypothesis was in fact entrusted by
him to his research associate, Anna Gillingham, who was a
psychologist. She was then joined by a teacher friend, Bessie
Stillman. Their joint work was eventually published under the
title, *Remedial Training for Children with Specific Disability in Reading,
Spelling and Penmanship*. The first edition appeared in 1946 and the
work has been revised many times. The quotations which follow
are drawn from the 1969 edition.

Gillingham and Stillman point out, early on in the book, that
besides the confusions in visual memory which had been so much

emphasized by Hinshelwood and Orton, there are in some cases confusions and reversals in recognizing and remembering *heard* words. For example, this was particularly pronounced in the case of a girl called Maud (pp. 5–6), whose two brothers, we are told, also had problems. When she attempted to express her ideas in speech this resulted in extreme mispronunciations, in failure to distinguish between /b/, /p/, /t/ and /d/ in repeating words and in inability to reproduce any vowel sounds clearly enough for them to be recognizable.

> A large part of Maud's training for a long period consisted in careful repetition of sounds made by the teacher and in forming associations between seen symbols and their sounds, between heard symbolic sounds and their appearance in print, between heard symbolic sounds and the feel in her hand as she wrote the corresponding letters.
>
> (Gillingham and Stillman 1969, p. 6)

Gillingham was of course familiar with Hinshelwood's book, and the teaching methods recommended are very similar to his in their basic principles.

> The technique in this book is based upon the constant use of association of all of the following – how a letter or word looks, how it sounds and how the speech organs or the hand in writing feels when producing it.
>
> (Gillingham and Stillman 1969, p. 17)

The writers were also familiar with the tracing procedures of Fernald (1943), whose book came out only three years before the first Gillingham–Stillman manual. It included various ways of introducing phonic teaching, though in Gillingham's view these were supplementary aids rather than part of an all-inclusive system, and were consequently inadequate. (In the later chapters, written by Stillman, there was a greater readiness to acknowledge a debt to Fernald.) For Gillingham, Orton's principles demanded a comprehensive method, involving close association of visual, auditory and kinaesthetic elements to form a 'language triangle'; to this end she devised procedures called 'linkages', which were to be used for the teaching of each new letter. These linkages are set out in full on pp. 40–2 of the manual. They can conveniently be summarized as follows:

1 The letter is shown and the child repeats the name after the teacher; when the name is known the sound is repeated in the same way.

2 The letter is written carefully by the teacher and its shape and orientation are explained; it is then traced over, copied, written from memory, and written again with the eyes averted.

3 The letter is shown and the child is asked to name it; his hand may be guided by the teacher, and he is asked to name it without looking. The name of the letter must be associated both with its 'look' and with its 'feel'.

4 The child is required to write the letter from dictation.

5 This is the same as 3, but with the sound asked for.

6 The name of the letter is given by the teacher and its sound is asked for.

7 The sound is given by the teacher and the name is asked for.

8 The sound is given by the teacher and the child is asked to write the appropriate letter, saying the name at the same time.

Then begins the process of teaching the child to build words from their sounds rather than to try to memorize them. During this process Gillingham insisted that the child should do no other reading elsewhere by a different approach. He has to learn a skill, and during this time interesting books can be read aloud to him.

There is a special routine for spelling, in which the teacher writes the word and reads it to the child; the child repeats it, then writes it naming the letters as he writes, then repeats the word once more. This is called Simultaneous Oral Spelling (SOS).

If Anna Gillingham seems harsh in her insistence on following this programme scrupulously, and not, for instance, making any attempt to find reading books that will interest the child, it is clear from the early pages of the manual that this is because she had seen the devastating effect of repeated failures at the hand of well-meaning teachers; she was determined to leave behind her a system that could not fail to produce literacy. Similarly she entrusted the continuation of her work to a former pupil whom she knew would be equally uncompromising, Sally Childs. She was right there; the latter was swift to say 'That's not Gillingham!' if she spotted the slightest deviation from the specified procedure. Those who had learnt from Anna Gillingham trusted her, because they knew how much the success obtained through her methods had meant to them.

The programme was, of course, produced at a time when 'look and say' methods were most in fashion; these are least suitable for the child who finds difficulty in mastering phoneme–

grapheme correspondence, in that they start with the most common words, and the most common words in English are of Anglo-Saxon origin, with irregular spelling patterns. Gillingham and Stillman were rebelling against this approach. Teachers experienced in teaching these children still maintain that a dyslexic pupil can master the alphabetic aspect of reading and writing only through a very systematic approach in which the child is progressively made aware of the correspondences between written symbols (both singly and in combination) and their sounds. In the words of another American dyslexia specialist, Margaret Rawson, the programme needs to be 'structured, sequential, cumulative, thorough, and multisensory'.

Another point that Gillingham makes is that children *enjoy* practice and discipline in acquiring skills, and any teacher who thinks otherwise is 'attributing her own attitude to the child' (Gillingham and Stillman 1969, p. 129). One has only to remember the popularity of groups such as majorettes and the enjoyment found in games like 'Simon Says' or 'Musical Statues' to see the shrewdness of this observation, especially in the case of small children.

However, the manual has much more than rigour to offer to the painstaking reader. In a later chapter, which Anna Gillingham says in the Foreword was one of those that were entirely Bessie Stillman's work, it is made clear that there are higher objectives than mere mechanical procedures; the manual speaks of the need to acquire a 'spelling sense'. For instance:

> We have stated as our goal the conversion of spelling into a thought subject whenever this is possible, meaning that we must so generalize and intellectualize the process as to provide a line of thought along which the confused speller can pass when all visual and auditory imagery of a word fails him. The lessons in generalizations are developed for the non-speller whose power of abstract thought can be enlisted to circumvent his unreliable visual recall.
>
> (Gillingham and Stillman 1969, p. 183)

Generalizations are important because they 'give a more fundamental training in thoughtful attack and foster a spelling sense and a feeling for English usage that do not come from merely applying rules' (p. 183).

There is, besides, much wise advice in the pages of the manual that is still relevant today.

The Gillingham–Stillman programme became a model for similar programmes both in the USA and in Great Britain. One of the best-known centres is that at the Scottish Rite Hospital in Dallas; and it was here that Sally Childs carried on Anna Gillingham's work, and was later succeeded by Aylett Cox. *Project Read* is one offshoot of the Gillingham programme, while Beth Slingerland developed a version of it for use in the classroom. In Great Britain the main progeny of the Gillingham–Stillman programme have been Kathleen Hickey's *A Language Training Course for Teachers and Learners* (Hickey 1977) and Bevé Hornsby and Frula Shear's *Alpha to Omega* (1975).

These two programmes have emerged as different in a number of ways. For Hickey, written language is the starting-point: 'The importance of the alphabet in education is that it is the basis of the English language' (1977, p. 14).

Gillingham had no particular reason for the order in which she introduced letters and their combinations other than that she did not wish to teach successively those letters which had two sounds or those letters which differed from each other merely in orientation. Nor did Hickey, although both she and Gillingham in fact started with vowels which were not easily confused in their short sounds, viz. 'a' and 'i'. Hickey, however, thought it important to introduce consonant blends as well, so as to provide a good choice of words to be built; she therefore introduces 's', 'n', 'p' and 't' early. With the introduction of 'd' she is able to give the word 'said' an early position. This is not because it relates in any way to the type of word being taught at the time; rather it is introduced in accordance with a principle which she follows throughout, viz. that words can be taught only if one has introduced all the constituent letters. Although Hickey shows a great deal of ingenuity in manipulating these combinations, one feels that she is not very much aware of the importance of choosing a vocabulary that a child most needs; thus she introduces 'stint', 'hasp' and 'bric-a-brac' right at the beginning. However, the Dyslexia Institute in using the programme have made modifications for their own use, and may in due course update it.

Hornsby and Shear (1975), as speech therapists, have a quite different starting-point. They are in no doubt that one should begin with the spoken language and build on it, and this principle pervades their whole work. By comparison Hickey's order seems less well planned, since she ignores the relationship between different consonant digraphs, such as 'th', 'sh' and 'ch', and between the double consonants that occur at the end of short vowels, such as '-ff', '-ss', '-ck', '-tch' and '-dge'. For Hickey, irregular words are taught as 'sight words', as they were by Gillingham and Stillman. Hornsby and Shear, however, have a definite policy of introducing them one or two at a time along with spelling patterns which give the same sound; for instance they introduce 'sword' and 'horde' when the 'or' pattern is being studied. This gives a definite oral basis at the start to which they can be attached; and one is therefore not just learning a meaningless string of letters. They also have an excellent system of grading the vocabulary according to frequency; this means that teachers can use their discretion, depending on the age and intelligence of the pupil, as to which words to introduce. Hornsby and Shear have the additional objective of teaching a developing language structure, starting with simple active affirmative declarative sentences and progressing gradually to more complex ones. The development in literary style does not, perhaps, quite match the laudable intentions, and the more elaborate sentences are sometimes unnatural and gauche, but the need for such training is fully recognized. Sometimes, too, in the early part of the book, a logical order is overstressed at the expense of word frequency, with the result that occasionally the book seems out of touch with classroom teaching – perhaps not surprisingly, since the authors were originally trained as speech therapists and not, like Hickey, as remedial teachers. For instance, single vowels have to be pursued to the end before the very common vowel digraphs, such as 'oo' and 'ee', are introduced at all, despite their frequency in young children's books; they do not in fact get a mention until after some 120 pages! The experienced teacher, however, knows well how to skip and adapt, and overall the book is an extremely useful one. As a companion to the programme there is a box of cards which are of a useful size for teaching purposes.

The *Bangor Dyslexia Teaching System* (E. Miles 1989) has only recently been published in full, but the Primary School stages have been in use by Bangor-trained teachers from 1978. The Secondary School stages were in due course added to form a distinct second part aimed at older children. It is a similar type of programme to the ones mentioned so far, although in fact it was not derived from the work of Gillingham and Stillman, but has been a British product from the beginning, having first been conceived in an attempt to help children referred to a Child Guidance Clinic in North Wales (Miles 1961). While having a very definite structure like the others, and taking note of linguistic features of the English spelling system, it is slightly more flexible and allows the teacher some choice of order. It gives very definite guidance on the differences in approach needed in teaching pupils of secondary rather than primary school age; prefixes and suffixes are studied in detail, and there is a section on study skills. Sentences are not included, but there is a stock of such sentences for pupils at the earlier stages in Miles and Miles (1983); after that teachers are expected to acquire for themselves the art of writing sentences which do not involve any spelling patterns not yet taught.

Another set of booklets recently published (Kingston Polytechnic 1985), but based on the Gillingham and Stillman approach, is that of the Kingston Learning Difficulties Project. There are separate reading and spelling packs, and the start is similar to that of the Gillingham–Stillman manual, though there is more emphasis on articulation. There are some useful work-sheets and games. The introduction of prefixes and suffixes in the first twenty pages and some sophisticated vocabulary in the first book ('bombastic', 'allocate') suggests that the work is not really intended for the young primary school child, and there is a suggestion that some of the pupils may already be able to read up to age level (p. iii), in which case the help is coming late. Most of the work-sheet material is simple enough, however, and the cursive writing style is attractive and clear. However, as in *Alpha to Omega*, some 100 pages pass before we are told anything about common vowel digraphs. There are other booklets on diagnosis, study skills and the special needs (in terms of enrichment) of able pupils in ordinary classrooms.

The *Spelling Made Easy* series of five books (Brand 1984) has narrower objectives, but is a multisensory structured spelling programme which, after offering 'family lists', gives dictations which enable the teacher to test a particular group of words. The final book, *Remedial Spelling*, is particularly distinctive from other programmes in presenting a range of spelling patterns up to a level needed by older students coming up to examination forms; and it gives passages of quite advanced vocabulary to test them, written in a reasonably flowing English style which approximates more to what is needed in their other school work.

All these programmes follow Hinshelwood and Orton in

finding value in a multisensory approach, some following more strict procedures than others. Brand (1984) could be speaking for all of them when she writes:

> Too much emphasis has been placed on learning to spell through visual methods. The ears and the mouth have been forgotten and the power of the hand ignored. If a child, or an adult, hears a sequence of sounds, sees them visually represented, feels the sequence in his mouth and reproduces the symbols with his hand, his awareness of the basis of written language is awakened. He feels that he can control it – and what he controls he can use.... The senses which they employ for normal communication, speech and hearing, are being involved in the written language which has previously defeated them.
>
> (Brand 1984, Level I, p. 3)

Gillingham and Stillman's *Simultaneous Oral Spelling* (see above for details) has also been found to be an extremely effective way of learning individual words (Bryant and Bradley 1985, pp. 130–6). As a check on this type of teaching in general, Hornsby and Miles (1980) examined the records kept at three centres specializing in dyslexia. They compared the pre-teaching rate of reading and spelling gain of over 100 children with the gains that they made during specialist teaching of the kind described above; the figures showed that in the case of over 80% of the children the contrast was striking.

There are other reasons too, of course, for a multisensory approach; if one is going to have to repeat the same material several times for it to be firmly fixed in the child's mind and become second nature, the only possible way to do so is to introduce every variety that the different modalities can offer. Children have to be interested to learn; they also have to be personally involved; and writing and speaking guarantee this in a way that merely looking and being talked to do not.

One final programme requires mention, viz. *Units of Sound* (Bramley 1984). This, too, is a very systematically organized and structured programme, with strong audio-visual links, since it has a set of 18 cassettes. While the sound unit is given at the top of the page, the emphasis is on reading whole words; the aim is to develop in the learner 'a recognition of pattern and rhyme involving visual, oral and auditory factors' (p. 6). Correct speech production, for example of 'th', is carefully explained or encouraged by example. Writing plays no part at the beginning, since recognition of and reading of the units of sound is the objective. Nevertheless the cassettes can be used for dictation afterwards so as to provide practice in the spelling of these units, and the lists of check words can be used as a foundation for practice sentences composed by the learners themselves. Explanation of the spelling points would, however, have to be filled in by the teacher. The vocabulary level and the readability level of the continuous passages rise, and the programme is designed in part for improvement in comprehension and to be acceptable to secondary school pupils and adults. It has puzzle questions at the end of a page requiring the pupil to find a word of that pattern with a particular meaning. Its great strength is its emphasis on individual learning, and it has great potential for teachers to use as an adjunct to personal teaching, where they can also pick and choose if they do not necessarily like Dr Bramley's way of presenting individual items. Thus Dr Bramley presents as units the combinations 'rn' (as in 'barn' and 'torn') and heads combinations such as 'a-e' at the top of the page simply with an 'a', whereas it is arguable that what is linguistically a correct description is not necessarily the most effective presentation for teaching.

There are also some aids to teaching which should receive mention, although they are not programmes in the full sense. These include the Edith Norrie Letter Case (see also Chapters 8 and 11), which relates letters to the place of articulation of their corresponding speech sounds, the Letterland version of Lyn Wendon's programme, which gives an exciting introduction to grapheme–phoneme correspondence for very young children, the *Aston Portfolio* (Aubrey *et al.* 1980), structured spelling books by Allan (1977, 1979), Pollock (1978) and Smelt (1976) a *Check List of Basic Sounds* Cotterell 1969), and *Phonic Reference Cards* (Cotterell 1975).

Both programmes and teaching aids contribute to the same purpose, which is that of remedying the phonological weaknesses of children with these specific difficulties (dyslexics) by the systematic building up of associations between speech sounds and their representations in writing.

11

Opponents and supporters of the dyslexia concept

It is clear that to many educationists the dyslexia concept came as a novel idea, and it was not easy for some of them to adjust to it. In Britain, at least, it is fair to say that the issue of dyslexia was largely ignored until the early 1960s, when the Invalid Children's Aid Association took the initiative in setting up the Word Blind Centre in north London. There was obvious interest in Scandinavia, as is shown by the work of Edith Norrie (late 1930s) and thereafter by Hallgren (see Chapter 4). In the USA the work initiated by Orton (see Chapter 1) was taken up, not indeed on a large scale, but in some locations with very considerable enthusiasm. These developments will be considered later in this chapter. In general, until the 1970s it was only a small minority of people who took the dyslexia concept seriously. One result of this has been that there are still many adults who now recognize themselves as dyslexic but who were not diagnosed as such in childhood.

The comments which follow are based largely on the authors' experience of the scene in Britain, though from their limited knowledge of the USA, Australia and New Zealand it would appear that there, too, the issues over 'recognizing' dyslexia have been largely similar.

In Britain the word 'dyslexia' first found its way into the legal system in the form of a reference to 'acute dyslexia' in the Chronically Sick and Disabled Persons Act, 1970, section 27. The word 'acute' was unfortunate, and appears simply to have been the result of slipshod drafting: presumably it is intended to mean

no more than 'severe', since 'coming sharply to a crisis', which is
the medical sense of 'acute', is clearly not applicable here. Be that
as it may, little notice was taken of this part of the Act; and the
next major step on the part of the Department of Education and
Science was to set up a Working Party. The outcome was the
Tizard Report, *Children with Specific Reading Difficulties* (Tizard
1972). Its conclusion was:

> We are highly sceptical of the view that a syndrome of 'develop-
> mental dyslexia' with a specific underlying cause and specific
> symptoms has been identified.... We think it would be better to
> adopt a more usefully descriptive term, 'specific reading diffi-
> culties', to describe the problems of the small group of children
> whose reading (and perhaps writing, spelling, and number)
> abilities are significantly below the standards which their abilities
> in other spheres would lead one to expect.
>
> (p. 3)

This was at least a start towards the recognition that there was a
problem of some kind.

Supporters of the dyslexia concept, however, were not slow to
point out that 'reading difficulties' (whether 'specific' or not) was
no satisfactory substitute for 'dyslexia' since, despite the passing
references to writing, spelling and number, the title of the report
called attention to reading only. Dyslexics, so they claimed, had
many other difficulties and indeed in some cases were reasonably
adequate readers; this meant that the emphasis on reading was
an inappropriate proposal for classification. The Bullock Report
(Bullock 1975) also contained a small number of references to
dyslexia, and it included a recognition that 'the problem of these
children can be chronic and severe' (p. 268). Surprisingly,
however, in view of the systematic research which had already
been carried out at the time of its publication, it asserted both in
the main text (p. 268) and the glossary (p. 587) that the term
dyslexia 'is not susceptible to precise operational definition'. No
reasons are given for this dogmatic statement. The great merit of
the Bullock Report, however, was that it tried to shift attention
away from reading to *language*, and its title, *A Language for Life*,
therefore makes an important contribution to educational
thinking in general.

The greatest step forward, however, came with the publication
of the Warnock Report (Warnock 1978). One of its main
proposals was to do away with all statutory 'categories of

handicap' and to speak instead of children with 'special educational needs'. Members of the committee estimated that up to 20% of all children would at some stage have one such need or another. From the point of view of dyslexia this recommendation was important, since supporters of the concept had continually complained, up to that point, that dyslexia was not one of the categories of handicap comparable with 'partially sighted', 'deaf', and so on; and if 'dyslexia' was to have been added there would have been the difficult problem of defining who was dyslexic in a legally watertight way. As it was, the Warnock Committee neatly side-stepped this problem, since, whatever the nature of dyslexia, no one could doubt that the children whom some people called 'dyslexic' had 'special needs'. When many of the recommendations of the Warnock Committee were implemented in the 1981 Education Act it became possible for a dyslexic child – no less than, for instance, a partially sighted child – to be 'statemented', that is, given a statement of 'special needs'. This was clearly a step forward.

Since, however, there was considerable uncertainty as to what should be official policy, the Department of Education and Science commissioned a review of relevant evidence. The result was a report (Tansley and Panckhurst 1981) which advocated use of the expression 'specific learning difficulties'. The authors' intention (p. 33) was to produce a term which could include the phenomena of dyslexia but did not carry the same theoretical commitment: the seriousness of the difficulties was not in dispute but the question of causation was left open. Shortly afterwards, a similar view was put forward by a Working Party of the Division of Educational and Child Psychology, a body which is affiliated to the British Psychological Society (see British Psychological Society 1983). The report contained an interesting summary of the earlier controversies and made a large number of recommendations. These were by no means hostile to the dyslexia concept even if not fully supportive. Recommendation II, 6, 3 on p. 19 may serve as a typical example:

> Parents and professional workers will no doubt continue to use the term 'dyslexia' and educational psychologists should accept that this is so, though they may wish to view the term only as a descriptive label, having no aetiological implications.

Although the wording is clearly intended to be conciliatory the implication is that there were some educational psychologists who regarded Critchley's (1970) concept of 'specific developmental dyslexia' as mistaken.

It remains for us to consider further some of the factors which have influenced those who have regarded themselves as opponents of the dyslexia concept. In what follows we propose to draw largely on our own personal experiences in discussion with teachers, educational administrators and educational psychologists.

On the basis of the evidence cited above it can be said that in the 1970s the reaction of the educational establishment to the concept of dyslexia was largely hostile and that in some quarters it continues to be so, even though, overall, this hostility is becoming less. In the case of educational psychologists, it is possible that they are not given adequate grounding in language disabilities on their training courses, and this may be the reason why the number of uncooperative ones remains relatively high.

One of the original reasons for this hostility seems to have been that the dyslexia concept came from medical specialists, who thus seemed to be encroaching on education's 'patch'. Until changes were made in the 1960s, the organization was such that there were uncomfortable overlaps between 'health' and 'education'; for example, mental handicap was treated as a medical matter rather than an educational one, and situations could arise in which Education Authorities consulted doctors on this matter even when psychologists had had more experience and training. Moreover it was possible for Medical Officers of Health to discover someone whom they believed to be dyslexic, to prescribe 'treatment' (the very word seemed inappropriate to educationists), and then expect the money to come from the education budget! It was also thought that doctors probably did not realize the complex pattern of differences to be found in the normal way in children's reading progress and that these could be understood without the seemingly esoteric term 'dyslexia'. Thus the mistakes alleged to be typical of 'dyslexics', such as confusion between 'b' and 'd', could be found in many children, and there was therefore no need to pick out a distinctive group. In addition it was sometimes supposed that if a child was labelled 'dyslexic' this implied some permanent disability and was therefore discouraging to remedial teachers. It was also suggested that 'dyslexia' was in effect no more than a name for our ignorance: people appeared to be defining it by exclusion – 'We will call this child "dyslexic" if we cannot find any other reason for his difficulties.'

Those who used the dyslexia concept were of course not intending to imply that nothing could be done to help – quite the contrary. This, however, was one of the misunderstandings current in the 1960s and 1970s. The view that one can define dyslexia only by 'exclusion' does not now seem tenable (see Chapter 6), but it has not wholly disappeared.

There was also a tendency, whenever this seemed plausible, to attribute children's reading and spelling difficulties to 'tensions within the home'. The argument was that if parental attitudes could be changed and/or the child's emotional problems be resolved then reading and spelling would automatically improve. This view is not widely held nowadays, though its influence is occasionally felt. Supporters of the dyslexia concept wished to say, instead, that if children showed behaviour problems these could in many cases be the consequence, not the cause, of their difficulties over literacy. It came to be realized that dyslexics needed help with much more than just reading and spelling: they needed to learn, for instance, how to organize their day, how to be sure of remembering appointments, how to use bus and train timetables, and much else. This was a recognition of the need (as some would put it) to treat 'the whole child' as opposed to treating some isolated weakness; and it became plain that, when the nature of the dyslexic handicap was understood, the tensions both within dyslexic individuals themselves and between them and their relatives were likely to become very much less.

Another source of irritation was that pressure to provide help for dyslexics regularly came from middle-class parents; and although this is not in fact surprising, since any pressure group on behalf of children is likely to comprise the more articulate parents, the impression was given that these parents wanted their children to receive special treatment and were trying to keep them separate for snobbish reasons – finding, so it seemed, a fashionable label by means of which they could conceal their child's all-round lack of ability and avoid the social stigma of having a child unable to follow in his parents' footsteps. Writing in the *Guardian* (30 December 1975) Crabtree, who at the time was a Lecturer in Education, expressed this irritation as follows: 'If you live in Acacia Avenue you are dyslexic; if you live in Gasworks Terrace you are thick.' It was seemingly the same attitude which led some parents to support the idea of grammar schools or to send their children away to boarding school. None of this has anything to do with the scientific value of the dyslexia concept, but issues that were logically quite different were not always distinguished.

An assumption that was sometimes made was that there is just one financial 'cake' of fixed size which must be equitably shared between slow learners, dyslexics, and anyone else with 'special needs'. It did not always occur to people that improvements were possible, for instance an increase of teacher awareness, at very modest cost; and it was not always appreciated that even from the point of view of 'value for money' it was uneconomic to allow children to sit at the back of the class learning nothing, quite apart from avoidable expenses in medical care or in treatment of the frustrated dyslexic who turns to crime.

It is possible, too, that some teachers, if they found that despite their best efforts a child failed to learn to read, may have supposed that this reflected on their competence; and such people may well have been reluctant to admit that there were ever any dyslexics in their classes! In fact, if a child is dyslexic, this implies that the teacher is *less* to blame rather than *more* to blame, but this was not always appreciated.

There were also emotional arguments against picking children out and 'labelling' them. These arguments were particularly frustrating to those who believed that, if only one were allowed to *identify* the children in question, then intensive use of the appropriate teaching procedures could transform their lives. On this view it would seem that if 'labelling' is forbidden the only option for a conscientious teacher is to try to give some unobtrusive help within the classroom, even though such a pussyfooting approach is much less likely to be successful. For some teachers the slogan of 'integration' even now seems to mean that it is morally wrong to withdraw a child from a classroom for any reason at all. This, however, is to assume that integration should always take the same form even when different children have widely different 'special needs'; and indeed it is sad to see a concept put forward by the Warnock Committee for quite different reasons being misused as though it implied the need for total uniformity. In our experience, if the problems of dyslexic children are tackled with sufficient determination in the primary school there will be no difficulty over their integration in the secondary school. As things are, it is only because these problems have *not* been tackled that withdrawal is necessary.

The proposed teaching methods were also criticized for their limited scope and objectives. A widely held view is that the 'dyslexia lobby' is insisting that children should simply be taught 'phonics' – dull exercises such as 'ker-ah-ter spells "cat"' – rather than being taught to 'read for meaning' and being encouraged to gain experience of 'real books'. What has tended to happen is that some experienced teachers, rightly reacting against an exclusively 'phonic' aproach in the initial teaching of reading, have assumed that nothing more is needed other than traditional 'good practice': either the dyslexia concept supports such 'good practice', they would argue, in which case it is unnecessary, or it advocates something different, in which case it is mistaken. What some of them may not have appreciated is that the objectives in helping a dyslexic child to read and spell are strictly limited, since the intention is to remedy particular weaknesses, not to propound a total teaching policy that is applicable in the case of all children. Given that a child has a deficiency at the phonological level it is surely 'good practice' to try to remedy this. There may, indeed, still be a few extremists who have seen phonics as the only answer for all children, with the rejection of all recent gains of understanding about the nature of reading; but there are 'all or nothing' advocates on all sides in education, not just in the dyslexia lobby.

Alongside the hostility, however, there was a striking growth, in different parts of the world, of organizations whose aim was to get the problems of the dyslexic properly recognized. It is these organizations that we must now mention.

First and foremost among such bodies has been the Orton Dyslexia Society (originally the 'Orton Society'), which was founded in the USA shortly after Orton's death in 1948. This society has branches throughout the United States, but is especially strong in certain areas, in particular in Dallas, where there is the Scottish Rite Hospital (see Chapter 10), in Michigan, which is the venue of 'Project Read', and in California, North Carolina, Florida, and the North-East. In 1974 the Society celebrated its first 25 years by inviting guests from many parts of the world; and both before and especially since that time it has been the acknowledged leader in the dyslexia field, bringing together experts from all disciplines to its annual November conference. Its journal, *The Bulletin of the Orton Society*, later renamed *Annals of Dyslexia*, disseminates in very readable form articles by both researchers and practitioners. More recently it has set up a brain bank to which dyslexics can bequeath their brains for post-mortem neurological examination (for reference to the work of Dr Albert Galaburda, of Harvard University, see Chapter 3).

In South Africa, Rebecca Oistrowick started work in the early 1950s, and was one of the pioneers who used multisensory methods. Today, although there is no official dyslexia organization in South Africa, the Rebecca Oistrowick School of Reading outside Johannesburg is a centre for assessment and advice.

The Word Blind Institute in Copenhagen began even earlier, in 1938, when Edith Norrie, on the basis of her own experience as a dyslexic, founded the first organization in the world devoted to diagnosing and teaching dyslexics, and made use of her ingenious Letter Case.

In Australia the visit of Dr Macdonald Critchley to Sydney in 1967 was the trigger for the start of SPELD (SPEcific Learning Difficulties) in New South Wales; the key figure here was Yvonne Stewart, who was afterwards awarded the AM (Australia Medal) for this work. Thereafter SPELD Victoria, SPELD South Australia, SPELD Queensland and SPELD Tasmania were founded, and after that associations were formed in Australian Central Territory, Northern Territory and Western Australia. SPELD NSW is still the largest association, and it does a remarkable job through its news-sheet in reviewing and distributing books. A few years later SPELD New Zealand was founded by Dr Jean Seabrook, who set up courses to train teachers to give private lessons in all parts of the country.

In Britain, meanwhile, several organizations had grown up. The earliest was at St Bartholomew's Hospital, where Maisie Holt, a psychologist, started teaching dyslexic children in 1960 at the instigation of Dr Alfred White Franklin, a paediatrician at the hospital who afterwards became Chairman of the Invalid Children's Aid Association (ICAA) (see below). Miss Holt took advice from Sally Childs, Anna Gillingham's successor in the USA (see Chapter 10), and developed a teaching approach which was similar to that of Gillingham and Stillman. This programme was further improved by her successor, Bevé Hornsby, who contributed the expertise of a speech therapist; it eventually developed into *Alpha to Omega* (Hornsby and Shear 1975). A clinic was set up which gave free help to large numbers of children and adults, paid for by the National Health Service. An offshoot of this is the Hornsby Centre in Wandsworth, and the Hornsby School which uses multisensory methods for all its children.

The Word Blind Centre in London was a short-term project established in 1963 under the auspices of the ICAA, mostly at Dr White Franklin's instigation. Its objective was to assess, study and teach children believed to be dyslexic in order to find out more about the nature of the condition. Details of the research carried out there will be found in Naidoo (1972). It was never intended that the project should be anything more than a short-term one, and the statement in the report of the Division of Educational and Child Psychology (British Psychological Society 1983, p. 11) that it closed 'because of lack of funds' is incorrect.

The closure of the Word Blind Centre in 1972 was the occasion for the expansion of several other centres, most of whose leaders had been involved in one way or another with the Word Blind Centre. The Helen Arkell Centre (1971) followed the rather more informal type of approach begun by Edith Norrie at the World Blind Institute in Copenhagen, where Helen Arkell herself trained. It is now based at Frensham, Surrey, where it offers a teaching service for dyslexics and courses for training teachers, including the Royal Society of Arts Diploma in 'Specific Learning Difficulties'. It has also been involved in running biennial Easter courses, mostly in Cambridge, which have been sponsored by the Linbury Trust. The Dyslexia Institute, which was started by the North Surrey Dyslexia Association in 1972 with Kathleen Hickey as the head teacher, has grown biggest of all. It now has some 21 institutes, 49 outposts and 36 school centres in England, Scotland and Guernsey. The Kathleen Hickey programme (see Chapter 10) is the one which is used. The present Director of Studies, Dr Harry Chasty, has done much to advance its stature. It has also done a considerable amount of teacher training, and has developed links with Crewe and Alsager College, Staffordshire, with Leicester University, and with Jordanhill College, Glasgow, in developing British Dyslexia Association and Royal Society of Arts Diploma courses. At the University College of North Wales, Bangor, from the mid-1960s, one of the present authors (T.R.M.) set up a unit which undertook assessments and carried out research, while a few years later the other author (E.M.) set up a peripatetic teaching service. Validated courses were developed for the training of teachers, and a course leading to an M.Ed. in the field of dyslexia was started in 1973. The Watford Dyslexia Unit, under Violet Brand, which began in 1982, provides cheap private lessons for large numbers of children in Hertfordshire schools; and Mrs Brand has been instrumental in starting up the Royal Society of Arts Diploma courses, both in the UK and in Australia. All the courses run by the above institutions have laid considerable stress on the need for trainee teachers to give tuition on an individual basis.

Of the other bodies which did important pioneering work in the field of dyslexia in Britain one of the earliest in the field was the unit at Aston University, founded by Dr Margaret Newton, who was co-author with Dr Michael Thomson of *The Aston Index* (Newton and Thomson 1976). Interesting work was also carried out by the Cambridge Specific Learning Disabilities Group, an organization which was largely the creation of Beryl Wattles and Professor Oliver Zangwill.

The British Dyslexia Association is the national organization and the parent body to which these other institutions are affiliated. It was founded in 1972 by Marion Welchman. Before this time she had helped to found the Bath Association for the Study of Dyslexia which ran courses for teachers under the direction of Sally Childs from the USA (see Chapter 10). Mrs Welchman recognized the need for a voluntary movement made up of local Dyslexia Associations which could then cover the whole country. In recent years the British Dyslexia Association has drawn on the advice of many professionals working in the field and has ensured that this advice is at the disposal of all members. It has also been able to liaise with the Department of Education and Science and to provide evidence and submissions to governmental committees. In addition it has been instrumental, through the Dyslexia Educational Trust, in obtaining funds to support teachers taking training courses provided by the various corporate members – something which has led to an increase in the teaching expertise throughout the country. From its headquarters in Reading it also runs an information and help-line service. At the time of writing there are over 70 affiliated local associations in England and Wales, and this testifies to the growing recognition of the dyslexic child's needs.

12

Outstanding disputes

In this final chapter we shall consider ways in which the views of opponents and supporters of the dyslexia concept can be brought together.

As we saw, some of the issues which seemed to be causing division were in fact based on misunderstanding. Thus it is accepted on all sides that children with so-called 'dyslexic' problems can be helped (in other words it is not a 'defeatist' label), and no one disputes that if a child has special needs every attempt should be made to meet these needs regardless of that child's social background. What we shall be concerned with in this final chapter is something rather different, viz. apparent points of dispute where there are genuine and valid arguments on both sides. In our view there are two main examples of this, though there may be others. In both cases what is involved is not so much disagreement as differences of emphasis.

These two examples can usefully be set out in the form of thesis and antithesis, as follows:

1 Dyslexia is a medical matter

   Dyslexia is an educational matter

2 Dyslexia is a unity

   Dyslexia is a diversity

The pressures which lead to these seemingly differing views can then be explored in such a way as to bring out their full significance.

1 *Medical or educational?*

There are those who assert, or sometimes assume, that 'dyslexia' is a 'medical' term. They then argue that because the help that is required is not medical but educational a description of the child as 'dyslexic' gives a misleading picture and should therefore be avoided.

What is not always appreciated is the relative lack of clear-cut rules by which one is entitled to assert that any term is or is not 'medical'. Clearly there is no dispute over standard cases: thus no one would wish to deny, for instance, that 'measles' and 'diabetes' are medical terms. There are other words, however, which belong in a 'grey' area, such as 'lame', 'depressed' and 'exhausted'; in these cases the implications are in part medical, in part not. As far as 'dyslexia' is concerned, the issue is to determine how far it functions (or should function) like a medical term and how far like an educational one. This can be done both by considering existing linguistic practice and by reflecting on what practices can usefully be advocated.

One way of exploring this matter is to consider how far other terms with 'medical' connotations can profitably be used in the case of 'dyslexia'. In particular it may be helpful to examine the terms 'patient', 'cure', 'diagnosis' and 'treatment'.

Many of us feel uneasy about describing developmental dyslexics as 'patients', and even if they become adequate readers and learn other 'coping' strategies we would most of us be reluctant to say that they had been 'cured'. 'Diagnosis', on the other hand, seems a perfectly proper expression. It is important to recognize, however, that it is used in many contexts other than medical ones. Thus psychologists can quite correctly be said to make 'diagnoses' when they draw conclusions from their assessments, while if a teacher decides, for instance, that the poor quality of a particular piece of work is due to the fact that the pupil was out late at a disco, this, too, can quite properly be described as a 'diagnosis'. Those who object to 'medical' terms may also like to note that it is quite common to speak of a garage mechanic as diagnosing a fault in someone's car and of a plumber as diagnosing faults in the water supply! As for 'treatment', it is interesting to note that in the Orton–Gillingham tradition teachers of dyslexics were regularly referred to as 'language therapists'; and this expression, though not everyone may wish to use it, at least has the merit of bringing out that a limitation at the phonological level is a disability in the sense of something which needs to be put right. The expression 'extra reading lessons from a remedial teacher' paints a very different picture and, in the opinion of many, a mistaken one.

In any case there are plenty of matters which belong both to medicine and to education. For instance, just because it may well be a doctor who first diagnoses a particular condition such as Down's syndrome it does not follow that psychologists or teachers have no part to play in helping the Down's syndrome child. In the case of dyslexia, although the help needed is educational it is quite possible to take up a 'medical' approach to the subject if one is interested, for instance, in anatomical research, cerebral dominance, or genetics. Critchley (1981, p. 2) went so far as to suggest that the doctor is the right person to make the initial diagnosis, but this view – which not surprisingly made him far from popular with educational psychologists – is not now accepted. There is a possible case for saying that a professional psychologist is the best person to make an 'official' diagnosis. At least in the straightforward cases, however, it is now clear that the presence of dyslexia will be obvious to anyone with the appropriate experience, whatever their 'paper' qualification; and it is more important that the diagnosis should be made than that people should spend time wrangling as to who should make it.

In general, there are reasons for emphasizing both the educational aspects of dyslexia and its medical aspects. Thus what may seem at first glance like a dispute over fundamentals may turn out to be no more than a difference of emphasis. It is not that the thesis is correct and the antithesis wrong, nor vice versa. The important thing is to be aware of all the reasons for regarding dyslexia as a medical matter and all the reasons for regarding it as an educational one. As a brief formulation, there is, in our view, a good case for saying that it is a medical matter in its origin and an educational matter in its treatment.

2 Unity or diversity?

The issue with regard to unity and diversity is not unlike that which arises between 'splitters' and 'lumpers' in botany; and, indeed, there are many situations for classificatory decision where one needs to ask, 'Do we want to stress similarities by classifying the phenomena under the same name or to stress differences by assigning different names?' Here, as in the earlier part of the chapter, the decision is one of where to place the emphasis. As far as dyslexia is concerned, it seems important not to emphasize one view at the expense of the other but to be aware of *all* the reasons for 'splitting' and *all* the reasons for 'lumping'.

The 'lumpers' *par excellence* are those who say that the manifestations of dyslexia constitute a syndrome or cluster of symptoms which belong together. The comments of Patterson (1981) in connection with syndromes of acquired dyslexia are relevant here: 'The patients assigned the same classification will indeed differ from one another, even in significant ways; but contrast them with a patient exemplifying another syndrome, and the differences between the first two patients will seem trivial.'

The main argument for 'lumping' is the clinical one. To those working in the dyslexia field there is an obvious unity despite the wide range of individual differences. It is possible for those with appropriate experience to say, with a high degree of confidence, 'A dyslexic child would (or would not) do that'; and it is a common finding in clinical practice that those diagnosed as dyslexic come to recognize that both their special skills and their distinctive difficulties form a coherent pattern. Particularly striking has been the experience of one of the present authors (T.R.M.) who has repeatedly been told, in connection with his books on dyslexia, that he has exactly described a particular child ('You might have been writing about our Johnny'). If 'dyslexia' – in the sense of an identifiable pattern of difficulties – was not in some sense a unity it is hard to see how such recognition could have taken place.

'Splitters', on the other hand, have claimed that dyslexia is not a 'single condition'. Underlying this claim appears to be the assumption that use of the expression 'single condition' implies that the phenomena are the outcome of a 'single cause'; thus the Tizard Committee considers the issue to be whether there is 'a syndrome of "developmental dyslexia" with a specific underlying cause' (Tizard 1972, p. 3). There is an important difference, however, between a 'single condition' and a diagnostic label. Few medical conditions for which there is a diagnostic label can usefully be called 'single', and questions of causation are often extremely complex. If the 'lumpers' are right in the case of dyslexia a diagnostic label is indeed necessary, but nothing follows from this about either a 'single condition' or a 'single cause'. In any case one of the advantages of the word 'syndrome' is that it can be used when one is aware that certain signs 'belong together' but is unaware of what is causing them.

The research described in Chapter 9 strongly suggests that a group of poor readers and spellers can be identified who show difficulties at the phonological level. It makes sense, therefore, to classify such people together on the grounds that the typical 'dyslexic signs' are the consequences of this initial phonological weakness. This does not preclude a large amount of variation. Thus suitable training may in some cases enable dyslexics to learn to read competently, and even spelling may reach a more or less adequate level; in other cases, however, the person may remain weak at both or in some cases weak at spelling only. With regard to other skills – mathematics, for example – there is likely to be even more variety, since success may well depend on what opportunities for training and self-improvement have been possible. It is often the case that dyslexics have 'missed out' on certain basics – recognition that subtraction sums should be started on the right, for instance, or that the number 'one hundred and three' should be written '103' and not, as a different logic might dictate, '1003'. It is not surprising, therefore, that some dyslexics acquire such skills while others do not. The fact that there is diversity does not preclude an underlying unity.

There is, however, a further problem for the 'lumpers'. If dyslexics constitute an identifiable group, then, as a matter of logic, it is necessary to specify criteria for membership of that group. In the straightforward cases this is not difficult; the 'classic signs' are available for anyone to see, and for research purposes appropriate specification of a suitable number of these signs, in the form of an operational definition, need not be a major source of difficulty. What is more problematic, however, is the issue of 'borderline cases'. Critchley and Critchley (1978) have suggested that there can be minor variants of dyslexia, which they call *formes frustes* and which they suggest are sometimes found in the relatives of more seriously affected persons. What is not clear is whether there is the possibility of a strict dividing line ('This person is dyslexic, this person is not') or whether the one shades into the other in such a way that any cut-off point is arbitrary. Both physical and social criteria may influence the decision here. According to social criteria one would count a person as 'dyslexic' only if his or her problems were serious enough to merit special attention; if, however, one were doing research into genetics it would clearly be wrong to ignore cases that from the educational point of view were very mild. It does not, of course, follow that the policy of 'lumping' is misguided; but there is a good case for saying that it is legitimate to draw different boundaries for different purposes. It is also a logical consequence of the 'lumping' policy that criteria need to be specified for distinguishing not only the reading-backward child from the underachieving (or 'reading-retarded' child) but for distinguishing dyslexic underachievers from other underachievers. Research involving this distinction has barely started.

Moreover, it is for these reasons that no satisfactory figures are available for the incidence of dyslexia in the narrow sense. From evidence supplied by Critchley (1970, pp. 94–6) and more recently by Tansley and Panckhurst (1981, pp. 163–84), and on the basis of unpublished data from the survey reported by Miles and Haslum (1986) it is possible to suggest a tentative figure of about 4 per cent, but the absence of consistent selection criteria makes the matter very much one of guesswork.

We suspect, overall, that the reasons for 'lumping' have not always been as well appreciated as the reasons for 'splitting'; and this has meant that differences between dyslexics have sometimes been stressed at the expense of similarities. The proper function of the word 'dyslexia', in our view, is to isolate a distinctive group of individuals and encourage a study of their characteristics and needs.

Suggestions for general reading

The following books cover a wide range of topics in the dyslexia field and also contain many further references:

Ellis, A.W. (1984). *Reading, Writing and Dyslexia*. London, Lawrence Erlbaum.

Hynd, G. and Cohen, M. (1983). *Dyslexia: Neuropsychological Theory, Research and Clinical Differentiation*. London and New York, Grune and Stratton.

Kamhi, A.G. and Catts, H.W. (1989). *Reading Disabilities. A Developmental Language Perspective*. Boston, Little Brown.

Pavlidis, G.Th. (ed.) (1990). *Perspectives on Dyslexia*, vols 1 and 2. Chichester, Wiley. (Published when the present book was in proof.)

Thomson, M.E. (1984). *Developmental Dyslexia*. London, Whurr.

References

Aaron, P.G., Phillips, S. and Larsen, S. (1988). Specific reading disability in historically famous persons. *J. Learning Disabil.*, **21**, 9, 521-84.

Allan, B.V. (1977). *Logical Spelling*. London, Collins.

Allan, B.V. (1979). *Spelling Patterns*. London, Collins.

Annett, M. (1985). *Left, Right, Hand and Brain: the Right Shift Theory*. London, Lawrence Erlbaum.

Annett, M. and Kilshaw, D. (1984). Lateral preference and skill in dyslexics: implications of the right shift theory. *J. Child Psychol. Psychiat.* **25**, 3, 357-77.

Aubrey, C., Eaves, J., Hicks, D. and Newton, M. (1980). *The Aston Portfolio*. Cambridge, Learning Development Aids.

Baddeley, A.D. (1976). *The Psychology of Memory*. London, Harper.

Baddeley, A.D. (1986). *Working Memory*. Oxford, Clarendon Press.

Baddeley, A.D., Ellis, N.C., Miles, T.R. and Lewis, V.J. (1982). Developmental and acquired dyslexia: a comparison. *Cognition*, **11**, 185-99.

Baddeley, A.D., Logie, R.H. and Ellis, N.C. (1988). Characteristics of developmental dyslexia. *Cognition*, **29**, 197-228.

Baddeley, A.D., Thomson, N. and Buchanan, M. (1975). Word length and the structure of short-term memory. *J. Verbal Learning and Verbal Behaviour*, **14**, 575-89.

Batty, S. (1986). Problems with dyslexia. In T.R. Miles and D.E. Gilroy, *Dyslexia at College*. London, Routledge.

Bishop, D.V.M. (1989). Unfixed reference, monocular occlusion, and developmental dyslexia - a critique. *Brit. J. Ophthalmol.*, **73**, 209-15.

Boder, E. (1973). Developmental dyslexia: a diagnostic approach based on three atypical reading-spelling patterns. *Develop. Med. Child Neurol.*, **15**, 663-87.

Bradley, L. and Bryant, P.E. (1978). Difficulties in auditory organisation as a possible cause of reading backwardness. *Nature*, **271**, 746-7.

Bradley, L. and Bryant, P.E. (1983). Categorising sounds and learning to read: a causal connection. *Nature*, **301**, 419–21.

Bramley, W. (1984). *Units of Sound*. Neston, Wilts., Units of Sound Productions.

Brand, V. (1984). *Spelling Made Easy*. Baldock, Egon.

British Psychological Society (1983). Specific learning difficulties: the 'specific reading difficulties' versus 'dyslexia' controversy resolved? *Occasional Papers*, **7**, 3.

Bryant, P.E. and Bradley, L. (1985). *Children's Reading Problems*. Oxford, Blackwell.

Bryant, P.E. and Impey, L. (1987). The similarities between normal readers and developmental and acquired dyslexics. *Cognition*, **24**, 121–37.

Bullock, A. (1975). *A Language for Life*. Report of the Committee of Inquiry appointed by the Secretary of State for Education and Science under the Chairmanship of Sir Alan Bullock FBA. London, HMSO.

Catts, H.W. (1989). Phonological processing deficits and reading disabilities. In A.G. Kamhi and H.W. Catts (eds) *Reading Disabilities: a Developmental Language Perspective*. Boston, Little, Brown.

Cheetham, J.S. and Ovenden, J.A. (1987). Tinted lens: hoax or help? *Australian J. Educ.*, **19**, 3, 10–12.

Coltheart, M., Patterson, K.E. and Marshall, J.C. (1986). (eds) *Deep Dyslexia*. London, Routledge and Kegan Paul.

Coltheart, M., Masterson, J., Byng, S., Prior, M. and Riddoch, J. (1983). Surface dyslexia. *Q.J.Exp. Psychol*, **25A**, 469–95.

Conrad, R. (1964). Acoustic confusion in immediate memory. *Brit. J. Psychol.*, **55**, 75–84.

Cotterell, G.C. (1969). *Check List of Basic Sounds*. Cambridge, Learning Development Aids.

Cotterell, G.C. (1975). *Phonic Reference Cards*. Cambridge, Learning Development Aids.

Critchley, M. (1970). *The Dyslexic Child*. London, Heinemann Medical Books.

Critchley, M. (1981). Dyslexia: an overview. In G.Th. Pavlidis and T.R. Miles (eds), *Dyslexia Research and its Applications to Education*. Chichester, Wiley.

Critchley, M. and Critchley, E.A. (1978). *Dyslexia Defined*. London, Heinemann Medical Books.

DeFries, J.C., Fulker, D.W. and LaBuda, M. (1987). Evidence for a genetic aetiology in reading disability twins. *Nature*, **329**, 537–9.

Denckla, M.B. and Rudel, R.G. (1976). Naming of object drawings by dyslexic and other learning disabled children. *Brain and Language*, **3**, 1–15.

Done, D.J. and Miles, T.R. (1978). Learning, memory, and dyslexia. In M.M. Gruneberg, P.E. Morris and R.N. Sykes (eds), *Practical Aspects of Memory*. London, Academic Press.

Done, D.J. and Miles, T.R. (1988). Age of word acquisition in developmental dyslexics as determined by response latencies in a picture naming task. In M.M. Gruneberg, P.E. Morris and R.N. Sykes (eds), *Practical Aspects of Memory: Current Research and Issues*, Vol. 2. Chichester, Wiley.

Duane, D. (1989). Neurobiological correlates of learning disorders. *American Academy of Child and Adolescent Psychiatry*, **28**, 3, 314–18.

Duffy, F.H., Denckla, M.B., McAnulty, G. and Holmes, J.A. (1988). Neurophysiological studies in dyslexia. In F. Plum (ed.), *Language, Communication, and the Brain*. New York, Raven Press.

Elliott, C.D., Murray, D.J. and Pearson, L.S. (1983). *The British Ability Scales*. Windsor, NFER-Nelson.

Ellis, A.W. (1984). *Reading, Writing, and Dyslexia: a Cognitive Analysis*. London, Lawrence Erlbaum.

Ellis, N.C. and Hennelly, R.A. (1980) A bilingual word-length effect: implications for intelligence testing and the relative ease of mental calculations in Welsh and English. *Brit. J. Psychol.*, **71**, 43–52.

Ellis, N.C. and Miles, T.R. (1977). Dyslexia as a limitation in the ability to process information. *Bull. Orton Soc.*, **27**, 72–81.

Fernald, G.M. (1943). *Remedial Techniques in Basic School Subjects*. New York, McGraw-Hill.

Finucci, J.M. and Childs, B. (1981). Are there really more dyslexic boys than girls? In A. Ansara, N. Geschwind, A. Galaburda, M. Albert and N. Gartrell (eds), *Sex Differences in Dyslexia*. Towson, Md., Orton Dyslexia Society.

Finucci, J.M., Guthrie, J.T., Childs, A.L., Abbey, H. and Childs, B. (1976). The genetics of specific reading disability. *Annals of Human Genetics*, **40**, 1–23.

Frith, U. (1985). Beneath the surface of developmental dyslexia. In K.E. Patterson, J.C. Marshall and M. Coltheart (eds), *Surface Dyslexia. Neuropsychological and Cognitive Studies of Phonological Reading*. London, Lawrence Erlbaum.

Galaburda, A.M. (1989). The brain of the dyslexic individual. Paper delivered at the conference of the Rodin Remediation Academy, Bangor, North Wales.

Galaburda, A.M., Corsiglia, J., Rosen, G.D. and Sherman, G.F. (1987). Planum temporale asymmetry: reappraisal since Geschwind and Levitsky. *Neuropsychologia*, **25**, 6, 853–68.

Geschwind, N. (1982). Why Orton was right. *Annals of Dyslexia*, **32**, 13–30.

Geschwind, N. and Behan, P. (1982). Left handedness: association with immune disease, migraine, and developmental learning disorder. *Proc. Nat. Acad. Sci., USA*, **79**, 5097–100.

Geschwind, N. and Levitsky, W. (1968). Human brain: left–right asymmetries in temporal speech region. *Science*, **161**, 186–7.

110   *Dyslexia: a hundred years on*

Gibson, J.J. (1968). *The Senses Considered as Perceptual Systems*. London, Allen
& Unwin.

Gillingham, A. and Stillman, B.E. (1969). *Remedial Training for Children with
Specific Disability in Reading, Spelling and Penmanship*. Cambridge, Mass.,
Educators Publishing Service.

Hallgren, B. (1950). Specific dyslexia (congenital word blindness). A
clinical and genetic study. *Acta Psychiatrica et Neurologica*, Supplementum
65, i–xi and 1–287.

Hampshire, S. (1981). *Susan's Story*. London, Sidgwick and Jackson.

Hartwig, L.J. (1984). One parent's experience with dyslexia. *Annals of
Dyslexia*, **34**, 313–18.

Head, H. (1926). *Aphasia and Kindred Disorders of Speech*. London, Macmillan.

Hermann, K. (1959). *Reading Disability. A Medical Study of Word-Blindness
and Related Handicaps*. Copenhagen, Munksgaard.

Hickey, K. (1977). *A Language Training Course for Teachers and Learners*.
London, Elizabeth Adams.

Hinshelwood, J. (1917). *Congenital Word-Blindness*. London, H.K. Lewis.

Hornsby, B. and Miles, T.R. (1980). The effects of a dyslexia-centred
teaching programme. *Brit. J. Educ. Psychol.*, **50**, 236–42.

Hornsby, B. and Shear, F. (1975). *Alpha to Omega*. London, Heinemann
Educational Books.

Howell, E. and Stanley, G. (1988). Colour and learning disability. *Clinical
and Experimental Optometry*, **71**, 2, 66–71.

Hubicki, M. (1990). Learning difficulties in music. Proceedings of the
International Conference on Dyslexia, organized by the British
Dyslexia Association and held in Bath (1989).

Hulme, C. (1981). *Reading Retardation and Multisensory Teaching*. London,
Routledge and Kegan Paul.

Hynd, G. and Cohen, M. (1983). *Dyslexia: Neuropsychological Theory,
Research, and Clinical Differentiation*. New York and London, Grune and
Stratton.

Jansons, K.M. (1988). A personal view of dyslexia and of thought
without language. In L. Weiskrantz (ed.) *Thought Without Language*.
Oxford, Oxford University Press.

Joffe, L.S. (1983). School mathematics and dyslexia: a matter of verbal
labelling, generalisation, horses and carts. *Cambridge Journal of Education*,
13, 3, 22–7.

Johnson, D.J. and Myklebust, H.R. (1967). *Learning Disabilities: Educational
Principles and Practices*. New York and London, Grune and Stratton.

Jorm, A.F. (1979). The cognitive and neurological basis of developmental
dyslexia: a theoretical framework and review. *Cognition*, **7**, 19–33.

Katz, R.B. (1986). Phonological deficiencies in children with reading
disability: evidence from an object-naming task. *Cognition*, **22**,
225–57.

Kingston Polytechnic (1985). Learning Difficulties Project Resource
Booklets.

Klopfer, B. and Kelley, D.M. (1943). *The Rorschach Technique.* New York, World Book Co.

Koffka, K. (1935). *Principles of Gestalt Psychology.* New York, Harcourt Brace.

Kussmaul, A. (1978). Word-deafness and word-blindness. In H. von Ziemssen (ed.), *Cyclopaedia of the Practice of Medicine,* Vol. 14 (Diseases of the nervous system and disturbances of speech). London, Sampson Row, Maston, Searle and Rivington.

LaBuda, M.C. and DeFries, J.C. (1988). Genetic and environmental etiologies of reading disability: a twin study. *Annals of Dyslexia,* **38,** 131–8.

Liberman, I.Y. (1983). Should so-called modality preferences determine the nature of instruction for children with reading disabilities? Paper delivered at the International Consortium on Dyslexia, Halkidiki, Greece.

Liberman, I.Y., Shankweiler, D., Fischer, F.W. and Carter, B. (1974). Explicit syllable and phoneme segmentation in the young child. *J. Exp. Child Psychol.,* **18,** 201–12.

Liberman, I.Y., Shankweiler, D., Orlando, C., Harris, K. and Bell-Berti, F. (1971). Letter confusions and reversals of sequence in the beginning reader: implications for Orton's theory of developmental dyslexia. *Cortex,* **7,** 127–42.

Lubs, H.A., Smith, S., Kimberling, W., Pennington, B., Gross-Glen, K. and Duara, R. (1988). In F. Plum (ed.), *Language, Communication, and the Brain.* New York, Raven Press.

McCarthy, J.J. and Kirk, S.A. (1961). *The Illinois Test of Psycholinguistic Abilities.* Urbana, Ill., Institute for Research in Exceptional Children.

MacMeeken, M. (1939). *Ocular Dominance in Relation to Developmental Aphasia.* London, University of London Press.

Marcel, A.J. (1986). Surface dyslexia and beginning reading: a revised hypothesis of the pronunciation of print and its impairments. In M. Coltheart, K.E. Patterson and J.C. Marshall (eds), *Deep Dyslexia.* London, Routledge and Kegan Paul.

Marshall, J.C. (1984). Rational taxonomy of developmental dyslexias. In R.N. Malatesha and H.A. Whitaker (eds), *Dyslexia: a Global Issue.* The Hague, Martinus Nijhoff.

Marshall, J.C. and Newcombe, F. (1973). Patterns of paralexia: a psycholinguistic approach. *J. Psycholinguist. Research,* **2,** 175–99.

Martin, S. (1986). Dyslexia in my life. In T.R. Miles and D.E. Gilroy, *Dyslexia at College.* London, Routledge.

Masland, R.L. (1976). The advantages of being dyslexic. *Bulletin of the Orton Society,* **26,** 10–18.

Mautner, T.S. (1984). Dyslexia – my invisible handicap. *Annals of Dyslexia,* **34,** 299–311.

Miles, E. (1989). *The Bangor Dyslexia Teaching System.* London, Whurr.

Miles, T.R. (1961). Two cases of developmental aphasia. *J. Child Psychol. Psychiat.*, **2**, 1, 48–70.

Miles, T.R. (1982). *The Bangor Dyslexia Test.* Cambridge, Learning Development Aids.

Miles, T.R. (1983. *Dyslexia: the Pattern of Difficulties.* Oxford, Blackwell.

Miles, T.R. (1986). On the persistence of dyslexic difficulties into adulthood. In G.Th. Pavlidis and D.F. Fisher (eds), *Dyslexia: its Neuropsychology and Treatment.* Chichester, Wiley.

Miles, T.R. (1987). *Understanding Dyslexia.* Bath, Bath Educational Publishers.

Miles, T.R. (1988). Counselling in dyslexia. *Counselling Psychology Quarterly*, **1**, 97–107.

Miles, T.R. and Ellis, N.C. (1981). A lexical encoding deficiency II: clinical observations. In G.Th. Pavlidis and T.R. Miles (eds), *Dyslexia Research and its Applications to Education.* Chichester, Wiley.

Miles, T.R. and Haslum, M.N. (1986). Dyslexia: anomaly or normal variation? *Annals of Dyslexia*, **36**, 103–17.

Miles, T.R. and Miles, E. (1983). *Help for Dyslexic Children.* London, Routledge.

Morgan, W.P. (1896). A case study of congenital word blindness. *Brit. Med. J.*, **2**, 1378.

Naidoo, S. (1972). *Specific Dyslexia.* London, Pitman.

Newman, S.P., Wadsworth, J.F., Archer, R. and Hockley, R. (1985). Ocular dominance, reading, and spelling ability in schoolchildren. *Brit. J. Ophthalmology*, **69**, 228–32.

Newton, M.J. and Thomson, M.E. (1976). *The Aston Index: a Classroom Test for Screening and Diagnosis of Language Difficulties.* Cambridge, Learning Development Aids.

O'Connor, P.D. and Sofo, F. (1988). A response to Gordon Stanley. *Australian J. Educ.*, **20**, 1, 10–12.

Oldfield, R.C. and Wingfield, A. (1965). Response latencies in naming objects. *Q.J.Exp. Psychol.*, **17**, 273–81.

Olson, R.K., Davidson, B.J., Kliegl, R. and Davies, S.E. (1984). Development of phonetic memory in disabled and normal readers. *J. Exp. Child Psychol.*, **37**, 187–206.

Orton, S.T. (1937). *Reading, Writing, and Speech Problems in Children.* New York, W.W. Norton.

Orton, S.T. (1966). *Word-Blindness in School Children and Other Papers on Strephosymbolia.* Pomfret, Conn., The Orton Society.

Patterson, K.E. (1981). Neurological approaches to the study of reading. *Brit. J. Psychol.*, **72**, 151–74.

Patterson, K.E. (1982). The relation between reading and phonological coding: further neurological observations. In A.W. Ellis (ed.), *Normality and Pathology in Cognitive Function.* London, Academic Press.

Pavlidis, G.Th. (1981). Sequencing, eye movements and the early objective diagnosis of dyslexia. In G.Th. Pavlidis and T.R. Miles (eds),

Dyslexia Research and its Applications to Education. Chichester, Wiley.

Peterson, R. (1987). A mother's story. *Australian J. Remed. Educ.*, **19**, 3, 12.

Pollock, J. (1978). *Signposts to Spelling.* Guildford, Helen Arkell Dyslexia Centre.

Pritchard, R.A., Miles, T.R., Chinn, S.J. and Taggart, A.T. (1989). Dyslexia and knowledge of number facts. *Links*, 14, 3, 17–20.

Quinault, F. (1972). Cross associations, opposites, and reversibility. University of St. Andrews: unpublished paper.

Rack, J.P. (1985). Orthographic and phonetic coding in developmental dyslexia. *Brit. J. Psychol.*, **76**, 325–40.

Raven, J.C. (1938). *Standard Progressive Matrices.* London, H.K. Lewis.

Raven, J.C. (1965). *Advanced Progressive Matrices.* London, H.K. Lewis.

Rawson, M.B. (1978). *Developmental Language Disability. Adult Accomplishments of Dyslexic Boys.* Cambridge, Mass., Educators Publishing Service.

Rawson, M.B. (1986). The many faces of dyslexia. *Annals of Dyslexia*, **36**, 179–91.

Rayner, K. (1986). Eye movements and the perceptual span. In G.Th. Pavlidis and D.F. Fisher (eds), *Dyslexia: its Neuropsychology and Treatment.* Chichester, Wiley.

Richards, I.L. (1985). *Dyslexia: a Study of Developmental and Maturational Factors Associated with a Specific Cognitive Profile.* Unpublished PhD thesis, University of Aston in Birmingham.

Richardson, S. (1989). Specific developmental dyslexia: retrospective and prospective views. *Annals of Dyslexia*, **39**, 3–23.

Robinson, G.L. and Miles, J. (1987). The use of coloured overlays to improve visual processing – a preliminary survey. *The Exceptional Child*, **34**, 1, 65–70.

Rugel, R.P. (1974). WISC sub-test scores of disabled readers. *J. Learning Disabil.*, **7**, 48–55.

Russell, W.R. and Espir, M.L.E. (1961). *Traumatic Aphasia. A Study of Aphasia in War Wounds of the Brain.* London, Oxford University Press.

Sartori, G., Barry, C. and Job, R. (1984). Phonological dyslexia: a review. In R.N. Malatesha and H.A. Whitaker (eds), *Dyslexia: a Global Issue.* The Hague, Martinus Nijhoff.

Seymour, P.H.K. (1986). *Cognitive Analysis of Dyslexia.* London, Routledge and Kegan Paul.

Simpson, E. (1980). *Reversals. A Personal Account of Victory over Dyslexia.* London, Gollancz.

Skinner, B.F. (1969). *Contingencies of Reinforcement.* Englewood Cliffs, NJ, Prentice-Hall.

Smelt, E.D. (1976). *Speak, Spell and Read English.* Victoria, Australia, Longman Cheshire.

Smith, P. (1988). *Music and Dyslexia.* London, Disabled Living Foundation.

Smith, S.D., Kimberling, W.J., Pennington, B.F. and Lubs, H.A. (1983). Specific reading disability: identification of an inherited form through linkage analysis. *Science*, **219**, 1345–7.

Snowling, M. (1987). *Dyslexia: a Cognitive Developmental Perspective*. Oxford, Blackwell.

Snowling, M., Goulandris, N., Bowlby, M. and Howell, P. (1986). Segmentation and speech perception in relation to reading skill: a developmental analysis. *J. Exp. Child Psychol.*, **41**, 489–507.

Spache, G.D. (1976). *Investigating the Issues of Reading Disabilities*. Boston, Allyn and Bacon.

Sperling, G. (1960). The information available in brief visual presentations. *Psychological Monographs*, **74**, No. 20.

Spring, C. and Capps, C. (1974). Encoding speed, rehearsal, and probed recall of dyslexic boys. *J. Educ. Psychol.*, **66**, 780–6.

Springer, S.P. and Deutsch, G. (1984). *Left Brain, Right Brain*. New York, W.H. Freeman.

Sprott, W.J.H. (1952). *Social Psychology*. London, Methuen.

Steeves, K.J. (1983). Memory as a factor in the computational efficiency of dyslexic children with high abstract reasoning ability. *Annals of Dyslexia*, **33**, 141–52.

Stein, J.F. (1989). Unfixed reference, monocular occlusion, and developmental dyslexia – a critique. *Brit. J. Ophthalmol.*, **73**, 319–20.

Stein, J.F. (1990). Unstable binocular control and poor visual direction sense in developmental dyslexics. Proceedings of the International Conference on Dyslexia, organized by the British Dyslexia Association, and held in Bath, 1989.

Stein, J.F. and Fowler, M.S. (1982). Diagnosis of dyslexia by means of a new indicator of eye dominance. *Brit. J. Ophthalmol.*, **66**, 332–6.

Stein, J.F. and Fowler, M.S. (1985). Effect of monocular occlusion on visuomotor perception and reading in dyslexic children. *The Lancet*, 13 July, 69–73.

Stein, N.L. (1987). Lost in the learning maze. *J. Learning Disabil.*, **20**, 409–10.

Stevenson, J., Graham, P., Fredman, G. and McLoughlin, V. (1987). A twin study of genetic influences on reading and spelling ability and disability. *J. Child Psychol. Psychiat.*, **28**, 2, 229–47.

Stewart, J.S.S. (1989). Some genetic aspects of dyslexia. Paper delivered at the conference of the Rodin Remediation Academy, Bangor, North Wales.

Stirling, E.G. and Miles, T.R. (1988). Naming ability and oral fluency in dyslexic adolescents. *Annals of Dyslexia*, **38**, 50–72.

Stuart, M. and Coltheart, M. (1988). Does reading develop in a sequence of stages? *Cognition*, **30**, 139–81.

Tallal, P. (1980). Auditory temporal perception, phonics, and reading disabilities in children. *Brain and Language*, **9**, 182–98.

Tallal, P. and Katz, W. (1989). Neuropsychological and neuroanatomical studies of developmental language/reading disorders. In C. von Euler, I. Lundberg and G. Lennerstrand (eds), *Brain and Reading*. Basingstoke, Macmillan.

Tallal, P. and Piercy, M. (1973). Developmental aphasia: impaired rate of non-verbal processing as a function of sensory modality. *Neuropsychologia*, **11**, 389-98.

Tansley, P. and Panckhurst, J. (1981). *Children with Specific Learning Difficulties: a Critical Review of Research*. Windsor, NFER-Nelson.

Taylor, J. (1931). *Selected Writings of John Hughlings Jackson* (edited). London, Staples Press.

Temple, C.M. (1985). Surface dyslexia: variations within a syndrome. In K.E. Patterson, J.C. Marshall and M. Coltheart (eds), *Surface Dyslexia*. London, Lawrence Erlbaum.

Temple, C.M. and Marshall, J.C. (1983). A case study of developmental phonological dyslexia. *Brit. J. Psychol.*, **74**, 517-33.

Terman, L.M. and Merrill, M.A. (1960). *Stanford-Binet Intelligence Scale*. London, Harrap.

Thomson, M.E. (1982). The assessment of children with specific reading difficulties (dyslexia) using the British Ability Scales. *Brit. J. Psychol.* **73**, 461-78.

Thomson, M.E. (1984). *Developmental Dyslexia*. London, Whurr.

Tizard, J. (1972). *Children with Specific Reading Difficulties* (Report of the Advisory Committee on Handicapped Children). London, HMSO.

Torgesen, J.K. and Houck, D.G. (1980). Processing deficiencies of learning-disabled children who perform poorly on the digit span test. *J. Educ. Psychol.*, **72**, 2, 141-60.

van den Bos, K.P. (1984). Letter processing in dyslexic subgroups. *Annals of Dyslexia*, **34**, 179-93.

Vellutino, F.R. (1979). *Dyslexia: Theory and Research*. Cambridge, Mass., MIT Press.

Vellutino, F.R. (1987). Dyslexia. *Scientific American*, **256**, 3, 20-7.

Vygotski, L. (1986). *Thought and Language* (trans. Alex Kozulin). Cambridge, Mass., MIT Press.

Warnock, M. (1978). *Special Educational Needs* (Report of the Committee of Enquiry into the Education of Handicapped Children and Young People). London, HMSO.

Wechsler, D. (1976). Wechsler Intelligence Scale for Children (WISC-R). New York, Psychological Corporation.

Whiting, P.R. (1988). Improvements in reading and other skills using Irlen coloured lenses. *Australian Journal of Remedial Education*, **20**, 1, 13-15.

Williams, A.L. and Miles, T.R. (1985). Rorschach responses of dyslexic children. *Annals of Dyslexia*, **35**, 51-66.

Wilsher, C.R. and Taylor, J.A. (1986). Remedies for dyslexia: proven or unproven? *Early Child Development and Care*, **27**, 287-99.

Winter, S. (1987). Irlen lenses: an appraisal. *The Australian Educational and Developmental Psychologist*, **4**, 2, 1–5.

Zangwill, O.L. and Blakemore, C.B. (1972). Dyslexia – reversal of eye movements during reading. *Neuropsychologia*, **10**, 371–5.

Index of names

Index of subjects

developmental aphasia vii
'dichotomania' 19
direct dyslexia 57
discrepancy vii, 36
dizygotic twins 25
Down's syndrome 102
Dunlop test 30
dyscalculia 48
dyslexia
  acquired 57–64
  as anomaly 42
  attentional 57
  auditory 50–6
  deep 57–64
  definition of by exclusion 93–4
  direct 57
  dyseidetic 53–4, 56
  dysphonetic 53–4
  exceptional talent in 40
  homogeneity of 102–5
  medical or educational? 100–2
  phonological 57–8, 61, 64
  surface 57–8, 61, 63–4
  as a syndrome vi–vii, 91, 103
  unity or diversity? 10, 102–5
  'visual' 30–2, 50–6
Dyslexia Educational Trust 99
Dyslexia Institute 85, 98
Dyslexia Unit, University College
  of North Wales 98
dysplasias 22

east–west confusion 40, 77
ecological validity 10
ectopias 22
Edith Norrie Letter Case 63, 89,
  97
Education Act, 1981 92
engrams 6
evolution, theory of 16–17
expressive language 45
eyedness 5, 19
eye movements 29

formes frustes of dyslexia 104

function words 58

genetics *see* heredity
Gestalten 53–4
Gestalt psychologists 7

handedness 5, 20–1, 38–9 *see also*
  laterality
handwriting 70
Haskins laboratories 65
Hawthorne effect 12–13, 68
Helen Arkell Dyslexia Centre 98
heredity, 5, 24–7, 104
Hornsby Dyslexia Centre 97

iconic memory 74
Illinois Test of Pshcholinguistic
  Abilities 52–3
imageable words 58–9
intelligence testing vii, 14, 42–3,
  46–7
Invalid Children's Aid Association
  90, 97
Irlen lenses 35–4

Japan, literacy in 77

kana 77
kanjis 77
kinetic reversals 6–8, 65

language triangle 82
laterality 19–21
left-handedness *see* handedness
left–right problems 38, 77
legasthenia vii
Letterland 89
lexicon, lexical entries 79
Linbury Trust 98
linkages 69, 82
logographic stage 69
long-term memory 73
'look and say' teaching methods
  13, 51, 83